MENTAL HEALTH CONSULTATION and EDUCATION

Arnold R. Beisser, M.D., Director
Center for Training in Community Psychiatry, Los Angeles

with

Rose Green, M.S.S., Professor Emeritus
School of Social Work, University of Southern California

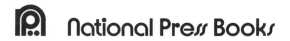 National Press Books

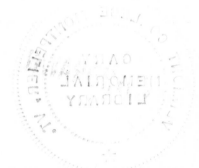

Book design by Nancy Sears

Library of Congress Catalog Card Number: 72-88950
International Standard Book Number: 0-87484-255-7
Manufactured in the United States of America

National Press Books, 850 Hansen Way, Palo Alto, California 94304

Dedicated to Jack and Helen Levin,
who are dedicated to each other,
to their family and legion of friends,
and to all things that may improve
the human condition.

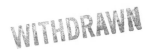

Contents

Preface

This book has been developed from seven years of teaching experience in the field of mental health consultation at the Center for Training in Community Psychiatry, in Los Angeles. More than two hundred professionals in psychology, psychiatry, social work, nursing, and related fields have participated in courses at the Center on this subject, and over the years they have helped to shape both the course content and the teaching methods presently used.

In writing this book, one of our major goals has been to meet the many requests for education in mental health consultation from areas with no access to such a program. These requests have come both from mental health groups and from colleges and universities throughout the country. In our text we have endeavored to reflect the Center's approach to education: while the book is a primer, it is to be used in a spirit of exploration, to serve as the basis on which a student or mental health consultant can learn new concepts and develop his unique skills.

We are fortunate to have had Rose Green as a faculty member

since the inception of the program. For thirty years Miss Green, Professor Emeritus of the School of Social Work at the University of Southern California, has been engaged in teaching consultation methods in the social work field. Her skills as an educator combine with her experience as a consultant to provide an uniquely comprehensive background. Miss Green has written chapters 5, 6, and 10. While the remainder of the work has been my responsibility, her inspiration and her cogent views have influenced the writing throughout, and it is with deep appreciation that I acknowledge her contribution to this work.

My own experience as a mental health consultant began in the early 1950's without the help of the currently available literature and without an experienced supervisor to guide me. I learned useful approaches from firsthand experience, but mostly I learned about the pitfalls. It was a powerful way of learning, but as a method it was more to my advantage than to that of the individuals and organizations with whom I worked. I hope that this book may help others to learn in ways which are less expensive to consultees.

For my own satisfaction it is necessary that the concept of mental health consultation described in this text encompass several areas to which I feel committed. My fundamental orientation is to the person centered, third force, humanistic psychotherapies. It has been necessary for me to attempt to integrate this with what I have learned from my experience in organizations both as a consultant and administrator. In addition, I have been strongly influenced by the scientific, analytic tradition and by my activities as an educator and group process facilitator. The concepts presented here are thus a personal and perhaps idiosyncratic blend of these varied involvements.

Many other faculty members have made significant conceptual contributions to this work. For example, Dr. S. Mark Doran was responsible for the establishment of consultation services for the Los Angeles County Mental Health Department, the largest such department in the world. We have drawn heavily on his experiences in developing working relationships in mental health consultation. Dr. Alexander S. Rogawski has added depth to the concept of group consultation with the "work family" in relation to theme interference. Dr. Janmeja Singh has incorporated a number of systems concepts into the theme interference model and has helped make it a practical approach. Drs. Irving Berkovitz, Donald Muhich, and Walter Brackelmanns have made contributions to our model by providing additional perspectives on schools and newly developing organizations.

Drs. Gerald Caplan and Portia Bell Hume have also made important contributions to this work. Dr. Caplan's concept of mental health consultation, which I have had occasion to discuss with him during periodic contacts since 1958, has served as a framework for testing experiences and focusing important issues. Dr. Hume's pioneering accomplishments in the development of mental health programs in California have provided me with essential opportunities in practice and teaching. Dr. Helen Olander, Associate Director of the Center for Training in Community Psychiatry, provided support and suggestions and acted as Director while I was on leave. Dr. Howard Parad also offered important suggestions and criticisms of the manuscript. Finally, Mrs. Daisy Johnson prepared the manuscript with the skills not only of a secretary but of an editor.

Special gratitude is due to the Levin Foundation and the Phillips Foundation, which made it possible for me to take time from my usual duties to prepare this manuscript. This support, provided through the Reiss-Davis Child Study Center, was secured through the efforts of Jack Levin, Helen Levin, Ing Backrack, Lester Deutsch, Jay Phillips, Samuel Maslon, and Dr. Rocco Motto. As with all of my other work, my wife Rita has helped in infinite, subtle, and essential ways.

Arnold R. Beisser
Los Angeles, California

Introduction to Mental Health Consultation

In his *History of Medical Psychology,* Gregory Zilboorg describes two psychiatric revolutions. The first reached its peak at the end of the eighteenth century during the Age of Reason. A transition took place in the prevailing concepts of deviance: those people who had been previously viewed as possessed by demons, willingly or unwillingly, became identified as "sick." This changed attitude and the related treatment accorded people had far-reaching effects on society. The symbolic political event of the era occurred when Phillipe Pinel struck off the chains from the inmates of the Bicêtre and Salpêtrière in France in 1793.

Zilboorg identifies a second psychiatric revolution at the end of the nineteenth century. The concept of mental illness had by then become consistent with the prevailing concept of physical disease. Cause-effect relationships were sought, and conscious behavior was found to be related to unconscious motivation. The personal life history of a patient became the equivalent of pathogenesis, with particular emphasis placed on the parent-child relationship. This extended the focus of concern to include the psychosocial environment. The great seminal figure of the period was Sigmund Freud, who systematized this emerging understanding in great detail.

A third psychiatric revolution, described by Leopold Bellak, took place in the mid-twentieth century. It was with the concept of community mental health, a logical extension of the preceding revolutions. If early family relationships were the cause of ensuing mental disorder, it was only logical to develop preventive measures within the potentially noxious context. If the stability and integrity of family life was related to the stability and integrity of the community and its organizations, it was a short step to begin to operate in the community arena as well. The third revolution, like the first, had its symbolic political act, when President John Kennedy called upon Congress for a "bold, new approach" to the treatment of mental illness. Congress responded by producing the most comprehensive mental health legislation in history, designed to produce two thousand mental health centers in the country by 1980 (Community Mental Health Centers Act, 1963).

Reflecting the prevailing public concerns of the period, psychiatry during the third revolution became oriented toward ecology; man could not be studied or treated in isolation, but had to be considered in intimate relation with his environment. Certain newly-considered aspects of the environment provided the field of psychiatry with a broader focus than before. Population growth, for example, had become exponential, so that, within living memory, where one person had stood there were now two or four. Moreover, this growth in actual numbers was made more apparent by the move from rural to urban life. The cities had grown at a rapid rate, pressing more and more people together into less and less space. At midcentury more than 80 percent of the population lived in cities — in contrast to only 25 percent of the population a century before. This population explosion and shift led to increasingly complex governing organizations and to a proliferation of the bureaucracies required for public service and order. As the family and communities ceded more and more of their functions to governmental resources, the development of service categories could not keep up with the need. People were alienated and often felt powerless to effect a change. Each intended solution seemed to carry with it the seeds of failure.

Each change to meet the problems of population growth and governmental complexity required additional change; the more things changed the more they were required to change. Organizational obsolescence became customary. With this ferment came a "communications explosion" which made constant awareness of environmental problems a fact of life. McLuhan likened this new awareness to that of a world-wide tribal community. The necessity for intervention on an ecological basis became readily apparent.

Even those who would confine themselves to a more traditional psychiatric practice were confronted by new research data from within the field. The optimism of the 1950s regarding psychotherapy as a means of dealing with all psychiatric and psychological disorders paled as these facts emerged. Massive epidemiologic studies showed that prevalence and incidence rates for mental and related disorders were so high as to preclude effective intervention by psychotherapy. The "Midtown Study" carried out in New York City, for example, showed rates remarkably similar to those of the Sterling County studies of small communities in the maritime provinces of Canada. Between 70 and 80 percent of the population in both areas showed some evidences of mental disorder and, even more startling, almost 25 percent showed the kinds of problems for which people entered mental hospitals. Other studies showed that the relationship between mental or emotional disorder and the provision of treatment was far less influenced by the degree of disorder than by issues of social class and ethnicity. In studies of psychiatric services in the New Haven area, for example, both the availability and the quality of treatment were found to be class-related. Clearly, there would never be enough psychotherapists to identify these problems, let alone deal with them. Just as clearly, some new sort of environmental intervention was necessary.

This raised a new issue, for it was impossible to identify the limits of responsibility for mental health professionals, who were operating in conjunction with a great many other specialized organizations and services. It was as though the community mental health movement were dedicated to the dissipation of its own categories of service. In a sense, this was the case, for one of the aims of community mental health was to go beyond established categories so that an individual in need of service could be helped without assuming a new and possibly incapacitating role.

Further, it was found that an organization dedicated to helping (such as a mental hospital) could in fact be unwittingly training its clients for incapacitation. Studies done within mental hospitals, clinics, and military establishments all documented that a patient's sacrifice of his autonomy for "help" could prove an incapacitating blow to his potential. Further studies of police records and of welfare, probation, public health, medical and legal agencies revealed that each had the same potential to incapacitate recipients of service. Clearly, environmental interventions were a necessity.

what can we do?

It is not enough merely to recognize the problem; practical methods for dealing with it must be devised. In the first revolution in psychiatry the sick were treated with compassion as people in need rather than as "possessed" and requiring punishment. "Moral treatment" was the therapeutic method which emerged. In the second revolution a detailed and elegant method was developed for intensive study and treatment of the individual in psychoanalysis. It carried with it a rational and scientific stance, reflective of the period, for application to human irrationality.

Some critics have said that there is no method of community psychiatric practice that can be taught. Others have complained that we simply "do not know enough" to prevent disorders. In answering this complaint, Caplan, in *Principles of Preventive Psychiatry,* has pointed out that the mental health professional of today knows a good deal more about the causes of disorder and its prevention than John Snow did, for example, at the time he intervened and interrupted the cholera epidemic of London, the prototypical event in the history of public health. His removal of the pump handle from the Broad Street pump was done without any knowledge of the vibrio cholerae or of the pathogenesis of cholera. It was based on a simple observation of the relationship between the use of the pump and the development of the disorder. At the very least, we know today that people seeking psychiatric treatment are, in part, the victims of an unhealthy environment: the communities and the organizations in which they live.

But what of the psychiatric method? In the early 1950s it appeared that crisis intervention, an approach based on identifying and helping at the point of maximum accessibility through psychotherapeutic means, might emerge as the core method of treatment. Indeed, its place in the scheme of community mental health is still of enormous importance. It has legitimized short-term intervention and has provided a framework for mental health workers to enter into a situation while it is still occurring.

Crisis intervention required only a modest reorientation of a mental health professional's traditional psychotherapeutic skills. It opened an acceptable alternative to long-term or intensive psychotherapy by helping people before they became identified as "patients." But as soon as responsibility is accepted for people who have not yet entered the treatment system, other approaches are required. Inevitably, work with people in crises leads to concern with ways in which organizations might provide the support and help necessary without the reorientation of role and the dislocation required in "becoming a patient." Thus studies of people in crisis have led to concern with organizational and community dynamics.

Emerging as the core method of community mental health is an approach which allows mental health professionals to reorient traditional psychotherapeutic skills while working with community organizations. The goal of this approach is often preventative. It seeks the maintenance of mental health while acknowledging the relationship of health to illness and pathogenesis. This is a necessary relationship to maintain so that the health professional can use what he already knows for the new purpose.

Mental health consultation is also appealing because in a period when the commotion of social change is dominant and social experience is tumultuous, it is a quiet method. It seeks to heal or prevent man/organization splits without the disruption characteristic of so many of the other methods of social change. Its purpose is to help people to cope with social systems as they are *now*, in a period of transition, rather than waiting for future changes to occur. It is a method which does not sacrifice the successful problem-solving of today for the changed environment of the future.

Mental health consultation is a conservative method in a period of radical methods. It is a balance and counter-force to the ever-accelerating pace of change. While it is a conservative method, mental health consultation nevertheless promotes integrative changes for workers, clients, and organizations. Although it seeks changes from the inside, it is a lubricant to whatever outside forces may require an organization to change. In short, it brings the knowledge and skills of mental health workers to bear on a turbulent social system.

roots of mental health consultation

Mental health consultation is a method which has emerged from clinical practice but also has roots in organizational theory and consultation. The experience and research derived from clinical practice has gradually led from a narrow physiological and psychological perspective on individual patients toward a social-systems approach focused on organizational dynamics and influences. The method combines elements of both, making it possible for a mental health professional to work within an organization toward mental health objectives.

By the mid-twentieth century there were many reports describing consultation in agencies. Such consultation was thought of as an extension of clinical psychiatric consultation. It was within the same model in which a specialist from any branch of medicine (e.g., surgery, cardiology, or dermatology) might consult with a general practitioner or specialist from another branch of medicine. Stedman's medical dictionary defines a consultant as a "physician or surgeon who does not take actual charge of a patient, but acts in an advisory capacity, deliberating with and counseling the personal attendant," and consultation as "a meeting of two or more physicians to consider the symptoms and the cause of the disease in any special case and to deliberate concerning the prognosis and the advisable therapeutic measures." This model, then, relied primarily on the consultant's personal interview with the client or patient and his recommendations to the person primarily responsible for the case.

Consultation in agencies with nonmedical personnel tended to follow this model. Almost always during the first half of this century the consultant had been a physician or psychiatrist. However, at midcentury, two types of changes had begun to take place. First, the consultants in agencies were no longer always psychiatrists. For example, often clinicians with backgrounds in psychology, nursing, and social work were utilized. The second change was even more significant. Consultants began to realize that problems did not always stem from ignorance or incompetence, but might have to do with some personal over-involvement in a case or with some of the pressures, problems, and policies within the agency. Thus, while the consultant was concerned with the client, it was also necessary for him to understand the system in which the client worked.

In 1947, Jules Coleman published the first paper dealing with mental health consultation in the form in which it is now practiced. Coleman's type of consultation was unique in that it focused not so much on the specific problem to be solved as on helping the consultee to deal with the case or client. The consultant attempted, in short, to assess what it was that interfered with the consultee's capacity to deal effectively with a case.

Of course the ultimate concern *is* the consultee's client. It was the assumption of Coleman and others that helping the consultee results in better service to the client. There have been fragmentary attempts to demonstrate this, but definitive research on the subject is yet to be done.

In 1950, Susselman described a working model, similar to the one elaborated by Coleman, in which attention was focused upon freeing the consultee of work problems and conflicts so as to increase his efficiency. In the same year Maddux described the use of Coleman's methods with public welfare workers. He was perhaps more specific in emphasizing that the consultant's task was to relieve the worker's anxiety or anger in order to increase his productivity. In the mid-1950s, Berlin also began reporting on his experiences as a mental health consultant. These reports utilized the same general approach as that described above. At about that same time reports of mental health consultation, with varying agencies and under differing circumstances, began to be prominent in the literature.

Gerald Caplan emerged during this period as the principle

figure and major conceptualizer. Drawing upon his own experience as well as the contributions of others, Caplan developed a method of mental health consultation which was both precise and practical. His theoretical formulation is so clear that in the past few years it has become the standard against which others measure their consultation activities. Differences and additions are noted in relationship to Caplan's model.

Caplan's description of theme interference and its reduction, perhaps because of its clarity and rigor, has been the subject of much controversy. Lydia Rapoport, for example, has summarized some of the differences and criticisms of the Caplan model in this way. "In essence, Dr. Caplan's methodology is anchored in certain assumptions and requires certain 'ideal' conditions, which are rarely obtained in the practice of consultation in social work—for example, that the consultant be an outsider to the consultee system; that the relationship be voluntary; that consultation be one-to-one rather than group consultation; that the supervisor or other intermediary not be present, unless he is the actual consultee; that the consultant be a skilled diagnostician and therapist who uses his knowledge, transferred and adapted, to deal with sensitive emotional blocks, essentially via the method of displacement, without getting into a therapeutic relationship, which would be a clear violation of the contract and intention."

She goes on to say that, in contrast to Dr. Caplan's model, most consultation is done in groups, in order to reach more people. She also finds insufficient attention paid to the "complex social system problems" which beset bureaucratic organizations and are reflected in staff turnover, low morale, and confusion of purpose. All are of high priority, especially as organizations are caught between conflicting social currents within the community.

She describes the Caplan model as "essentially an elitist model of consultation," in a period when many mental health professionals with limited training and experience are called upon to do consultation, and when consultees of marginal competence and experience sometimes face overwhelming problems. Nevertheless, the field of consultation is deeply in Dr. Caplan's debt for the classic clarity and precision of his descriptions.

If indeed the social-systems issues are the most pressing, the consultant working within an agency must broaden his understanding of organizational and management theory and practice. The most useful model would be one utilizing the knowledge and skills derived from clinical practice combined with the knowledge and skills derived from organizational and management activities.

twentieth-century organizational and management concept

The major model in the first half of the twentieth century emphasized the structure of an organization, with its principal ordering agency the bureaucracy. It was originally developed by Max Weber, both for efficiency and humane purpose. The model was developed as a reaction to the personal subjugation, nepotism, cruelty, emotional vicissitudes, and subjective judgment which passed for managerial practices early in the Industrial Revolution, and in the German army. The model emphasized rules and regulations, rationality, predictability, specialization, a well-defined hierarchy of authority, all to the end of making it an impersonal system of interpersonal relationships. The assumption was that if the personal factor could be removed, human irrationality would be limited, and equality of opportunity, justice, and efficiency would prevail.

Consultation, in this early period of organizational and management theory, was designed entirely for increasing efficiency in the accomplishment of the task. Frederick Taylor, an American engineer, was the first important organizational consultant employing what he called "scientific management." But "Taylorism," which focused on work measurement and analysis and on technology, increasingly sacrificed the worker to the task. What was developed by Weber for humane purpose became, in part, an instrument for social repression in the scientific management era.

The major failure of scientific management consultation was that it treated man's personality and social needs as either constant or nonexistent. However, personal needs and responses inevitably crept into organizational processes in unsuspected ways, and had to be dealt with. Informal organizations arose within the formal structure to serve these needs.

Understandably, there were hostile reactions to the impersonal bureaucratic model and especially the "scientific management" form of consultation. As a result of this backlash the human relations-oriented consultant came into prominence. He thought it impossible to ignore the attitudes, feelings and desires of workers, and his major assumption was that if a man's social and psychological needs were fulfilled he would work more productively. Thus, in the famous Hawthorne researches, Roethlisberger and Dickson focused their efforts entirely on workers' feelings, attitudes, beliefs, perceptions, and ideas.

With this interest in individual attitudes came an increased awareness of the significance of group attitudes and dynamics. A sense of group involvement, with resultant higher morale, was thought to be important to worker efficiency. Other consultation methods were based on the work of Mayo, Lewin, and Rogers, directed toward the satisfaction of both the individual and the group in work activities.

By midcentury, the limitations of both the scientific-management and the human-relations approaches had become apparent, and a new body of consultation experience began to emerge, causing revision of some of the more extravagant claims of human-relations theorists and yet maintaining a major concern for the individual and groups working in an organization. This consultation approach focused on man-organization conflicts, acknowledging the existence of organizational power issues and conflicting role responsibilities and granting the indispensability of the concept of authority. Thus a consultation model evolved which focused not only on the task and individuals involved, but also on group relations, role responsibilities, and formal and informal organizational structures. Consultants attempted to bring together in problem-solving groups the people who were actually involved in trying to perform the task. The interfaces between hierarchical levels and horizontal groups were bridged through various kinds of group meetings and communicative efforts, including "T" groups.

As the rate of social change increased, organizational consultants were faced with trying to bring organizations developed with outmoded methods for obsolete purposes into effective relationship with a rapidly changing environment. Consultants to organizations within this model became agents for change. They had to deal with the integration of changes in personnel, role definition, tasks and procedures. The methods used ranged from the small-group to the giant sociotechnical-systems approaches.

The knowledge and experience gained from these organizational consultation experiences are relevant to the consultation activities of mental health professionals. The agencies to which a mental health consultant provides services are undergoing precisely the same kinds of stress encountered and described by the organizational and management consultants.

What can the mental health consultant learn from the organizational consultant that will be useful to him in his consultations to service agencies? Perhaps the most important concept to be learned by the mental health consultant is that of the interdependence of individual workers, groups, and subsystems in any organization. By understanding the components of the social system and the ways in which they interact, the mental health professional is better prepared to deal with certain of these issues. Some of the issues to which he must attend are the task and the limitations imposed by regulation in the performance of the task, the lines of authority, the management practices—formal and informal—within the organization, intragroup dynamics, the dynamics between groups having different or overlapping responsibilities within the organization, and the preparation of individuals to perform their given tasks.

There are, however, significant differences between mental health consultation and organizational development consultation. Although there is some overlap, confusion may arise because of these differences. To begin with, the mental health consultant usually represents a program the goals and purpose of which relate to the treatment and prevention of mental disorder. When the mental health consultant goes to work in another organization, he does so carrying with him the goals and purposes of his own program. To some extent the consultee organization shares these goals. In such social welfare areas as probation, public health, and education, this common concern is very extensive.

The organizational consultant to industry has a somewhat different purpose. He is usually hired as an individual by an industrial organization specifically to improve its efficiency and productivity. While the consultant focuses on the needs and emotional responses of the workers, his major goal is to increase their output of work or perhaps to get them to perceive organizational goals more clearly.

The mental health consultant enters the organization with a concern for the whole person. The breadth of this concern may, in itself, create certain problems as he is tempted to ignore the organizational structure and purposes because of his concern for the person he meets. From his psychotherapeutic training he is prepared to go with whatever his consultee or client sees as an important problem. This may take him away from the consultee's role and task in the organization.

The agencies to which a mental health consultant offers services are concerned with helping people, but that help is limited by the organizational structure and goals. The mental health consultant has usually been trained as a psychotherapist and as such is committed to allowing a client or patient complete freedom in the focus of their work together. However, in his consultant's role he must be alert to maintaining the focus prescribed by the contract and the organization's goals. The danger lies in dealing with the consultee's problem outside of the organizational context, and possibly helping the consultee to be a more fulfilled person, but at the expense of reducing his effectiveness to deal with the needs of his client.

In order to avoid this, the consultant must continue to focus on the realities of the task and role of the worker. This is a major transition in focus for the mental health professional who has been trained as a psychotherapist concerned not with a segment of the person he works with but with his whole being and his entire spectrum of satisfactions.

Yet industrial consultation has increasingly come to realize that it must focus on the reality of the human desires and feelings of workers lest they become lost in the technology and work against the organization's efficiency. The consultant coming from the mental health field must work with a highly focused task and see human desires and feelings as related to that task. It is this challenge which creates the majority of problems for the mental health professional entering into consultation with an organization.

The industrial organizational consultant has learned to enter the organization by studying the total social system: its purposes, its methods, its structure, its processes, and its roles and those who fill the roles. The mental health professional has, from his therapeutic training, learned to study the whole person or self system. The mental health consultant has the task of bringing his special knowledge of the self system to bear on understanding of the social system.

teaching mental health consultation

In 1965, the Center for Training in Community Psychiatry opened in Los Angeles. One of its purposes was to provide training in mental health consultation to the professionals offering such services. With the emergence of new legislation at the state (California, 1958 and 1969) and federal (Community Mental Health Centers Act, 1963), levels, comprehensive mental health programs—reflecting the third psychiatric revolution—were developing. The professionals working in such programs had not been trained fully, except in their clinical work. They were called upon to provide mental health consultation, usually with a minimum amount of training and experience.

By 1972 the Center had given training to approximately two hundred mental health professionals and had developed a considerable body of experience in conducting this training. The Center staff learned a good deal about the kinds of problems faced by mental health professionals in the transition from the role of direct service clinician to mental health consultant.

Initially, trainees were carefully selected and limited to experienced clinicians from social work, psychiatry, psychology, and nursing. However, even among experienced clinicians, the diversity of perspective and wide range of background and experience presented problems. The center sought to provide training that built on existing skills and concepts held by trainees. Yet this building process was difficult in view of the range of differences among the experienced professionals.

The problem was further complicated by an increasing recognition of the fact that many of the people providing mental health consultation and representing mental health programs were *not* experienced clinicians. Rather, they were sometimes marginally trained and inexperienced, and sometimes came from outside fields such as education and sociology. The question facing the Center was whether to continue an elitist training program for those who already had extensive credentials, or to attempt the much more difficult and perhaps impossible task of providing training for the broad range of individuals who were actually providing services. The latter and more difficult course was chosen.

Out of this experience a model has been developed at the Center which draws heavily upon the model described by Gerald Caplan but draws equally on consultation experiences gained from industry and elsewhere. The model is deliberately broad, with minimal theoretical elaboration. Theory has been spared wherever possible, in the service of a practical approach by which persons of different theoretical persuasion may add to their backgrounds and skill in mental health consultation.

In a single small group of trainees at the center, for example, were a psychiatrist who was a Freudian psychoanalyst, a psychiatrist who was a Jungian analyst, a psychologist whose background and central interest were in learning theory and behavior modification, a social worker whose orientation was toward process, a psychologist who was a Gestalt therapist, and a nurse with training in several of the above approaches. In other groups, there were an educational psychologist who had been in charge of a mental health center's consultation program, a priest who was a psychologist, and a man with major experience in organizational consultation. With this in mind one can see the importance of having a generic model. Although our model is consistent with concepts of unconscious motivation, these are not usually explicitly used. Only where absolutely necessary are such theoretical issues raised; instead, the focus is on the practical performance of the task at hand.

In summary, then, the model to be described here is the product of collaborative study among a variety of people with a wide range of backgrounds. It is representative not only of the Center faculty but of all those who have participated in the Center's educational program.

The model described is presented in a linear fashion, as though consultation actually proceeds in the given sequence. It is presented in this way to serve as a guide to the consultant. It should be recognized, however, that each consultation may start at a different stage. Moreover, the sequence of stages may sometimes vary, and there may be periods of regression when an initial phase of consultation and the problems faced by the consultant during that period will emerge again at a later period.

The most important ingredient for learning mental health consultation is a commitment to the process of learning itself. Wearied from long educational experience, mental health professionals are often reluctant to commit themselves to learning a new process. The alternative of needing to discover all knowledge and skill *de novo* is hardly appealing, nor is it consistent with the urgency of the mental health needs within the community.

This primer has been designed to build on the mental health worker's already existing skills in order to make it possible for professionals from a variety of settings and backgrounds to engage in a combination of guided and self-directed study in order to help fulfill those urgent needs within the community.

CHAPTER I

A Primer and Study Guide

1. **What is this book?**

   This book is a primer for mental health consultants. Its goal is to present briefly and succinctly the principles of mental health consultation and education. It contains exercises so that both beginning and experienced consultants can practice the material described in the text.

2. **For whom is it written?**

   It is written for the beginner and will be especially useful to psychiatrists, psychologists, social workers, nurses, and others who are performing mental health consultation functions. It is assumed that the prospective consultant has a basic background in one of these mental health specialties which will serve as the basis for his work. This book attempts to focus the knowledge and skills of clinical work into an organizational perspective providing an approach whereby mental health workers can assist other service workers to be more effective.

3. How is it organized?

The text is organized in the form of a dialogue between student and teacher. The questions and points raised by the student are representative of those which are most pressing to students of mental health consultation. The purpose of this technique is to make the reading as lively and practical as possible.

Following the text of each lesson is a group of exercises and simulations which illustrate the points made. Each exercise relates to one or more of the questions in the text so that the student can refer to the text when discussing the experience of the exercise.

4. How should it be used?

An individual student may read the text and, in the exercises, imagine himself in the various parts, using the book as one would any other primer. However, it is best for two or more students to work on the book together. The text should be read carefully and individually by the participants. When they have finished, they should discuss the points, making certain that they understand them. Then they should begin the exercises. By breaking into smaller groups, an unlimited number of students can work together on the exercises. In the first few exercises it is well to work in small groups as described. If the total number of students is large, in later sessions it is well to have at least one or two of the exercises performed as a demonstration before the group.

After each exercise, at least a few minutes should be spent in discussing the experience. At this time it is well to have a discussion leader for timekeeping and focusing purposes. Preferably, this person should be a mental health consultant experienced and trained in the method described. However, an experienced teacher or group leader can also be effective.

We suggest that the discussion focus on the experience of the participants as much as possible. Analysis and criticism are of greatest value when based on the solid experience of those involved. While the roles are simulated, the students will find that they quickly get into them and are involved as fully as if they were actually in consultation.

We also suggest that a regular time be set aside for the study of the text and the exercises. The following plan has been used effectively by the authors.

Each week the text for the following week is distributed to

the participants. Sessions are organized into three-hour periods. After having read the text during the week, the participants discuss it for the first hour and a half of the session. Questions are raised and issues considered. After a fifteen-minute break, the exercises are performed for an hour. The last fifteen minutes of the three-hour period is devoted to a summary of the major points.

After the first few lessons, the group may find it useful to alter the format so that the exercises precede the discussion. This brings live data and experience into the session at the beginning.

Following each chapter there are usually more exercises than can be performed in an hour. Exercises can be selected based on points in the text which are ambiguous or problematic.

5. **What is the theoretical orientation of the primer?**

The theoretical material is kept to a minimum. Insofar as possible, this book is a practical guide, a "how to do it" book. Inevitably, the conceptual biases of the authors are present, and when this is the case they are made explicit.

The material can be best described as "process-oriented." That is, it is descriptive of the transactional and interactional processes necessary to effective consultation. This orientation is compatible with most of the contemporary frames of reference in the American mental health field. A single exception may be the approach of behavior modification, since this approach usually has a single measurable outcome for which the consultee is "trained."

6. **How would you characterize the conceptual framework beyond its being process-oriented?**

Our model emphasizes the freedom of the consultee to accept, reject, or modify what he learns from consultation. It emphasizes an egalitarian spirit between consultant and consultee. That is, it emphasizes that the consultation process takes place between two workers, each competent to do his job. In our model each must respect the competence and ability of the other as well as the organizational goals of the mental health program and the consultee program.

In addition, our model is task-focused. The anchor point is in the immediate job of the consultee: the service to be provided to a welfare recipient, a probationee, or to a public school student.

Our model is a mental *health* model, focusing on the enhancement of strengths and potential of the consultee to do the job, rather than a mental *illness* model, focusing on deficiencies. The consultant's efforts are directed to strengthen the capacity and interest of the consultee in doing his job.

7. Who should be a mental health consultant?

The term "consultant" implies an expert in his field. Thus, ideally, the mental health consultant should be an experienced clinician from one of the mental health clinical fields, such as psychiatry, psychology, social work, or nursing. The clinician who has integrated fragments of knowledge of his field and who has a firm identity as a professional clinician will find it easiest to move toward being a mental health consultant.

However, the reality is that many professionals are required to perform mental health consultation functions before they are seasoned clinicians. In these days of crash programs and accelerated learning, when the needs are so great, those who have just been certified in their professions, and many whose qualifications in the mental health field are incomplete, are required to offer mental health consultation. This guide has been written to be of use to a wide range of mental health workers from varying backgrounds. Even widely experienced consultants may find it useful.

8. Which organizations need a mental health consultant?

Organizations which usually employ mental health consultants are schools, welfare agencies, probation departments, health departments, police departments, groups of ministers, rehabilitation agencies, and other professionals providing human services. But mental health consultation has its use in any agency that seeks to help people in some way. Mental health consultation activities have been reported with bartenders, beauty parlor operators, political groups, and an almost infinite variety of other kinds of workers.

9. Which agencies within a community should have priority in providing mental health consultation?

Priority usually results from two factors:

A. The mental health consultant's services are first offered to those agencies which are in the best position to prevent mental disorder. Most mental health programs have such priorities in preliminary epidemiology and community organization studies.

B. Priority is often given to those agencies in the community who request such services. Such requests may come because an agency is new, in turmoil, or seeking to be more responsive. They may be initiated by workers who are having difficulty with clients, or administrators who are responding to new or changing program demands.

10. **Is it, then, a task-oriented method that can be used with anyone who has a role and a task to do?**

In a sense that is true. The model can be used effectively wherever anyone has a formally defined work role with tasks. The principal area in which the model has been tested has been in organizations which provide services such as those described above. However, it could be used whenever someone is responsible for working with others.

---

exercises for chapter 1

1. Each member of the group should take a couple of minutes to report his name, discipline, the agency in which he works, what kind of activities he carries out in his job, and what his interest in studying mental health consultation is. If the group is larger than twenty-five, it should be broken into smaller groups for this activity. If the group is composed of members of the same agency who are well acquainted, only the question regarding interest may need an answer.

2. Now break into groups of four. Ideally, groups should consist of members who do not know each other. Each member of each group should tell in a few minutes of an experience in which he

has received consultation. Afterward the group members should discuss:

1) What things they found useful in the experience of being a consultee and what was not useful.

2) What things did they like and not like about being a consultee.

3. Now return to the large group. Select a discussion leader. Each group should report on what it learned about the experience of being a consultee: what was useful and what was not.

4. Now break into groups by *discipline* (psychiatrists, social workers, nurses, psychologists, etc.). Each group should consider in what specific areas its members can serve as a consultant; that is, "In what am I an expert?" Consider this question from the standpoint of what in your training qualifies you as an expert for what kinds of problems and what categories of consultees. Be as specific as possible in terms of your knowledge and skills. Each discipline group should then make a single list of the areas of knowledge and skills which it has that could be useful in consultation.

The papers should be posted together on the wall so that each member of the total group can compare the disciplines listed. The entire group should then reconvene, select a leader and spend about ten minutes in discussing similarities and differences among the disciplines.

5. Now each person should individually list the areas and skills in which he is qualified as an expert. These areas may be related to his disciplinary training, other special training, or special life experiences. Each participant's list should then be posted on the wall. Members should browse among them for about twenty minutes. Then select a leader for the whole group for discussion of what was noted. Discussion should focus on differences and similarities of qualifications.

CHAPTER 2

The Structure of Mental Health Consultation

1. **What is the purpose of mental health consultation within a community mental health program?**

   Mental health consultation is an integral part of a comprehensive mental health program. It is, in fact, a required component of the program in federally supported community mental health centers. It is meant to perform the following functions:

   A. To improve the mental health climate of other organizations and agencies so as to promote the healthy functioning of their clients (primary prevention).

   B. To strengthen and improve the capacity of workers in other organizations, such as schools, welfare agencies, and public health organizations, to handle effectively the human and emotional crises of their clients (secondary prevention).

   C. To facilitate the recovery, with as few crippling effects as possible, of those who have suffered mental or emotional disorder. By enhancement of the supportive climate and acceptance of patients and former patients in the community and its agencies, rehabilitation is furthered and the risk of future breakdown reduced (tertiary prevention).

2. What are the definitional characteristics of mental health consultation?

A. Who is involved in mental health consultation?

The *consultant* is a mental health professional skilled in the clinical application of services to those with mental and emotional disorders. Usually he is from one of the generic mental health professions, i.e., psychiatry, psychology, social work, or nursing.

The *consultee* is an individual or group of individuals working in an agency or organization in the community dealing with specialized needs of people. The primary purpose of these workers is not provision of mental health services, but because of their contact with people there is a mental health element in their work. Examples are schoolteachers, ministers, job supervisors, social welfare workers, and probation workers.

B. What is the subject of mental health consultation?

The subject of mental health consultation is the mental health aspect of the consultee's work. It may relate to individual clients, a group of clients, or the program objectives and structure of the consultee's agency. Consultation is usually organized around a current work problem identified by the consultee, or it may be related to future planning within an agency.

C. Where is mental health consultation held?

Usually it is held in the consultee's agency so that the life space and context of the subject of the consultation may be observed and taken into account.

D. When is it held?

It is held at the initiation of the consultee. This may be on an ad hoc basis, at regular intervals, or for a time-limited period. The frequency and intensity of the sessions depend on the needs of the consultee and the availability of the consultant's time.

3. What are the goals of mental health consultation?

A. The first goal is the *primum non nocere*, that is, to do no harm. Because knowledge of clinical psychopathology is a potent force, the mental health consultant must be constantly vigilant that he does not leave the consultee less able to function effectively and supportively with his clients than before, because he has become doubtful of his abilities or preoccupied with his own mental health problems.

B. The second goal is to strengthen the capacity, interest, and confidence of the consultee in carrying out the mental health element of his job. The focus, then, is more on the *healthy* functioning of the consultee and his clients than it is in the usual clinical setting, where the focus is on "what's wrong" with the patient and on his ineffective behavior. While clearly, "what's wrong" and "what's right" with someone's functioning are parts of a whole, this focus on *health* orientation may represent a significant shift for some mental health professionals.

4. **How is mental health consultation different from other forms of consultation?**

   A. *Consultation between members of the same discipline:* When a professional is having difficulty with some aspect of his work he may call upon a senior member of his profession for consultation and advice. For example, a physician may call in a senior colleague to consider cases not going well. This form of consultation is different from a mental health consultation in several ways. The consultee asks the Consultant, "What's wrong?" in the case and, since they share the same basic background and professional responsibilities, he calls upon the authority and wisdom of the consultant to tell him what he should do differently.

   By contrast, in mental health consultation, consultee and consultant are from different disciplines with different responsibilities. They must form a coordinate relationship, each having approximately equal amounts to contribute to the solution of the problem. While the consultant may be an expert in mental health, he is probably not an expert in school education or the ministry. Each must help the other to learn about his system and its relevance to the case at hand.

B. *Technical assistance:* The consultant is requested to develop a plan for dealing with a particular issue. The consultant does the "job" himself and the agency is dependent upon him for it. Specialized knowledge or skill is called upon for design and/or implementation of a task within the organization.

In mental health consultation the consultant attempts to *strengthen* the independent functioning of the consultee. The consultant's contribution to the agency's work is only through the staff's increased effectiveness. Consultant and consultee work together as equals on a task of *common* concern: the health of the community and its individuals. The consultee, however, retains responsibility for the work they consider together.

C. *Organizational development:* A consultant may be hired as a "change agent" to facilitate a change in the organizational structure or function. Such consultation usually occurs in a human relations model in industry or private agencies which are either small enough or autonomous enough to allow for such planned change to occur.

Mental health consultation usually occurs within large public agencies. The organizational structure and functions of workers within the agency are usually prescribed by law and code. This limits the authority of the organization and staff to make changes. Therefore the process in mental health consultation is to facilitate the functioning of workers *within* the structure as it is.

Of course, this distinction is not so arbitrary as it may appear at first. Public agencies can and do change from inside and private agencies and small agencies are not so free to change as may appear on the surface. However overdrawn the arbitrary distinctions may be, it is important to keep them in mind while determining what the organization wishes.

5. What are the characteristics of this coordinate relationship?

A. Each must respect the other's *competence* to do the job

he is carrying out. The consultant must assume that the worker has the professional skills and knowledge to carry out the tasks assigned to him by the agency. He must assume that he is not competent to judge the professional performance of the consultee, and that this is the task of the consultee's supervisor and administrator.

B. The consultant must *respect* the organizational and disciplinary goals of the consultee organization and *respect* their competence to carry them out. If he does not, he is likely to become a saboteur, attempting to "right" the errors of the agency or to act as a "change agent," which would be inappropriate to his function.

C. *Interdependence:* The mental health consultant, representing the mental health organization, has a stake in the functioning of the consultee organization in its promotion of mental health and its potential for reduction of mental illness. He is dependent upon the good will and acceptance of consultees to promote these ends.

In dealing with an individual case or problem, the consultant is dependent upon the consultee for the initiation of the discussion, for an accurate description of not only the case but the structural and organizational constraints in the case and the prescribed role responsibilities and limits which he has in the organization. The consultee relies upon the consultant for understanding of both the case and the consultee within the context of his work, and for the addition of a mental health perspective in the work.

6. How is the social context of mental health consultation unique?

Mental health consultation is a process which occurs at the interface between two organizational systems.

A. The consultant is responsible to his mental health program.

B. The consultee is responsible to the program in which he works: e.g., public health, social welfare, probation, schools, etc.

These differing responsibilities must be an explicit part of discussions and negotiations which occur between consultant and consultee.

7. **What are the responsibilities of the consultant and consultee?**

   A. The consultee is responsible for any action which occurs as a result of the consultation. He is free to accept, reject, modify, or distort what comes out of the consultation process.

   B. The consultant is responsible for the consultation process. He must try to make it a constructive effort, insofar as he has control over it, consistent with the mental health principles he knows.

8. **Does this really mean that the consultant has no responsibility for a destructive act which develops from consultation?**

   The consultant may find that there are results which he cannot approve. In that case he may choose to relinquish the consultation role, but he should be aware of the effect of this action on future consultation.

   While he may have initiated the idea of consultation, the consultant has been called in at the *invitation* of the consultee organization. He is a guest, without the rights and responsibilities of an organization member.

9. **How is mental health consultation different from other related services and activities in the mental health field?**

   A. Clinical services.

      1) *Psychotherapy: Mental health consultation is to work role as psychotherapy is to self.* The consultant should view the discussion through the limited window of the consultee's work role as he defines it. The consultee presents a problem with a client, not a problem with himself. He asks for assistance to do his job better, not for improving his personality or reducing his symptoms. The consultant must accept and support this focus and if the consultee begins to move toward self-exploration, the consultant must refocus the consultation on role activities.

      By contrast, the patient presents *himself* as the problem. He does not say, "Help me to do my job better," or, "How do I deal with this troublesome client?" but, "I have a problem." The psychotherapist accepts this definition and accepts the patient as someone who needs help with himself.

2) *Case work:* Case work deals with a selected function of the self, sometimes in carrying out a particular task. It sometimes is in relationship to providing tangible resources such as money or housing. But again the focus is on the person and on his inability to function effectively within a particular context. The case work client presents *himself* as the problem.

3) *Sensitivity training:* Sensitivity training employs group and individual methods in a relatively unselected way to enhance the sensitivity, understanding, and communication of participants. It is usually carried out without an organizational context and seeks deliberately to reduce the role concerns of participants. Groups are usually composed of strangers who have elected to join together to enhance their human understanding in a general way outside of organizational or work context. In fact, this freedom from organizational constraint is often considered an essential part of effective sensitivity training.

B. Intraorganizational functions.

1) *Supervision:* The supervisor provides services to the supervisee which may, in many respects, resemble consultation. However, he retains responsibility for the case in question as well as the work performance of the supervisee. The supervisor's responsibilities include judgment of the worker's competence. It is on his recommendation, for example, that the worker receives merit salary increases and promotions. However cordial the relationship between supervisor and supervisee, this authority and responsibility are irreducible components of the relationship and distinguish it from consultation.

2) *Administration:* Closely linked to supervision, administration retains ultimate authority and responsibility for the activities within an organization. The administrator must establish standards and work allocations. He, too, may develop warm working relationships with others in the organization

but ultimately he is responsible for the agency's activities.

C. Interorganizational functions.

    1) *Liaison:* The mental health worker may serve as a liaison person between organizations in the community. He opens communication channels, provides and receives information, and represents the mental health program. He is not responsible for a helping task in an organization outside his own except as a by-product of his liaison activities.

    2) *Negotiation:* Representing the mental health program, a professional may find himself negotiating with other community agencies — often the ones with which he later becomes involved as a mental health consultant. Negotiation may relate to the establishment of common procedures: for example, the method of screening the consultee agencies' clients for referral to the mental health program. In fact, before the mental health consultant begins his consultation activities he must negotiate on behalf of his own organization with the consultee organization for the privileges and activities which he will be carrying out.

    3) *Collaboration:* A mental health professional may also work in collaboration with other agencies and their workers — often those for whom he may at some point become a consultant. Each has responsibilities for a portion of the work associated with a case or a client. For example, the mental health program may provide a child with psychotherapy while the school provides education. It may be useful for the workers in these two programs to communicate about their progress.

D. Extraorganizational functions.

    1) *Community organization:* The mental health professional may play an important role in developing community relationships for the mental health program and in determining community need for services. His goal may be to develop community support for his program.

    2) *Community development:* Mental health profes-

sionals may assist communities to develop their own resources to answer needs, instead of relating them in some way to services offered by existing agencies. Such efforts occur within indigenous community groups and outside the structure of existing service organizations.

3) *Social action:* While community organization and development may both be seen as forms of social action, the term has in large part become synonymous with confrontation technique. In this form the mental health professional may be hired by or join with a community group to bring pressure on a community service facility to alter its operations in some way. In this sense, social action is at the opposite pole from mental health consultation. It seeks to bring change by outside pressure, while the mental health consultant works "within the system." It is important for the mental health professional to distinguish for himself in which of these activities he is playing a part.

If he is to serve the organization as a mental health consultant, he must respect its goals and competence to achieve them. If he enters an organization as a mental health consultant but with a secret desire for social action, he may prove himself destructive to the organization and to the various services which he hopes to improve. On the other hand, if he enters as a mental health consultant, he may find himself quite unwelcome in a social action group.

---

exercises for chapter 2

1. A. Individually, think of a current work problem which you would feel free to discuss with your supervisor.
    B. Think of a current work problem which you would not feel free to discuss with your supervisor.

C. Break into groups of four, each composed of some of the different disciplines present. Discuss with the other group members the problems you have thought of, focusing on the kinds of things which are appropriate and comfortable to discuss with a supervisor and those which are not.

2. Pair off with someone from the same discipline. Think of a practical problem related to your discipline, and then discuss the problem for five minutes with your colleague as though he were your consultant. Following that, discuss with your colleague what each of you had hoped to get from the consultation.

3. Change partners, this time working with someone from another discipline. Individually think of a case you are working with clinically that involves another social service organization, such as a school system or welfare department. As a pair, then choose one of the two cases suggested. The person who suggested the case takes the role of the mental health clinician, and the other the role of the schoolteacher or caseworker. The mental health professional then initiates a five-minute consultation with the other about the client. Afterwards, discuss what happened from the standpoint of:
   A. What each member wanted from the consultation.
   B. What working relationship each member wanted with the other person.
   C. What each member wanted to avoid in the consultation.
   D. The process of the consultation.

4. This time silently think about a professional (for example, a minister, lawyer, doctor, or schoolteacher) from another field whom you know who is having trouble with a client. If necessary, invent a problem. Now play this role in a five-minute consultation with your partner as a mental health professional. After you are finished, discuss what each member wanted and did not want from the consultation.

5. Together think over the simulated consultations in exercises 3 and 4. Did you have the impression that the other person treated you as though you were competent, and with respect? Did you feel

that it was an egalitarian and interdependent relationship, or was there a feeling that a subordinate was requesting something of a superior?

6. Individually, think of a social agency, some aspects of whose functioning you do not respect. Now think of the means you might use to change them. Think of how your trying to change this would affect the administrator and the workers. How would your efforts affect services offered consumers?

    Now join into groups of four and discuss your thoughts. Consider the impact on the system of your efforts to influence and change.

7. Silently think of a professional person in another field whose work you respect and whom you consider competent. Imagine that person coming to you with a mental health problem concerning a client. What would you have to offer and what would he expect? Now turn to your group and discuss.

8. Following are a series of statements describing problems presented by consultees. Think about the kinds of comments you would make which would focus on "what's wrong" (the pathological aspect) in the situation presented. Then think about the kinds of responses which would focus on "what's right" (the healthy aspect).

    A. A teacher discusses a child who clings to her, won't go outside for recess, and does everything possible to try to be close to her.

    Suggestion: "What's wrong:" You don't seem to like dependence.

    "What's right:" You would like so much for him to be able to take care of himself.

    B. A public health nurse talks about the fact that she would like to transfer a case of a man who is dying because she feels she is too involved in the case.

    C. An unmarried welfare worker describes, as though she were annoyed, a mother with four children who has just become pregnant by an unknown man.

    D. A probation officer discusses one of his charges who is on probation for exhibitionism and who he believes is exhibiting himself but not telling the probation worker.

In each case, enact the consultation. After each simulation discuss the experience.

9. Join into new groups of four, this time simulating the interface between two social systems. One person will play a consultant, the second his administrator in a mental health program, the third a schoolteacher, and the fourth the school principal.

   First, the representatives of the mental health program discuss together what the goals of the program are, the administrator laying out what he expects for the total program as well as this consultation. The schoolteacher and principal discuss the goals of the school and objectives for students, and then discuss what they hope will develop from consultation. The teacher and the mental health consultant then meet, their respective administrators sitting behind them. Periodically each considers with his administrator what is happening in the consultation. The case is of a junior high school girl of high academic potential who is failing. Her work dropped off a year ago after her parents separated. Enact the consultation.

10. Now, continuing in these same pairings, see what happens when the mental health consultant tries to take responsibility for the student. See what happens when the schoolteacher tries to abdicate her responsibility for the girl. Reenact the consultation.

CHAPTER 3

The Context of
Mental Health Consultation

1. **What is the situational context of mental health consultation?**

    Mental health consultation takes place at the interface of two social systems: the consultant system (mental health) and the consultee system (schools, social welfare, public health, probation, etc.).

2. **Why emphasize the social systems? Isn't the important interaction the one between consultant and consultee?**

    Of course, but the consultant and consultee operate within fields of influence which determine their interaction. If these fields are forgotten or ignored, the consultation is likely to be irrelevant or destructive.

3. **Why is that?**

    The consultee works in an organization with rules and values that are unique to it. Similarly, the consultant brings with him the rules of his mental health program and the values of the mental health field. If the consultation is only a two-person interaction, as it is in psychotherapy, for example, the consultee may find that what he has gotten from the experience is at odds with or cannot be translated into the tasks, rules, and resources of his agency. If the consultant forgets the goals, rules, and resources of his program, he may find himself overcommitting his time or his program's time and doing things not in keeping with his program's objectives. Moreover, if the consultant and consultee are supported by community groups or tax revenue, they will not be doing what they are hired to do if they ignore the contextual field.

Consultation is a potent intervention and either it may help the consultee to work effectively or it may make him more dissatisfied, less effective, and counter-productive in the organization. The latter is likely to occur if the system's issues have been ignored. Mental health consultation is not isolated from the social context and may cause reverberations throughout the system.

4. **Does that mean that the consultant has to accept all of the negative things he sees in the system?**

It is not for the consultant to accept or reject the components of the system. Rather, each component represents a piece of data which must be included in any adequate solution to a problem presented. Otherwise, in dealing with one problem, he may create several more.

5. **But after all, isn't there good evidence that all of these systems — schools, probation, health, welfare, and the ministry — are in trouble, are changing, and need to be changed further?**

Yes. All of these institutions are in change, but mental health consultation is concerned with what can be done *now*. It is a method designed to help the workers in these unstable systems to work effectively for their clients and public so that a generation of them need not be sacrificed while we bring about change.

6. **What does the consultant need to know about the social systems?**

Let's conceptualize it this way:

The circles all overlap at the point of interface. Let's assume that the large circle on the left is the mental health system — made up of the network of service programs, professionals, clients, and patients. Each of these is a subsystem.

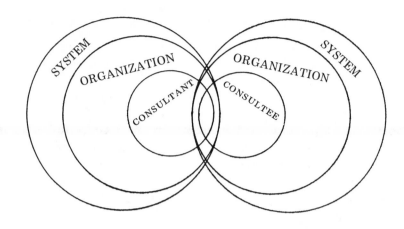

The large circle on the right represents the consultee system. It, too, is made up of a group of subsystems: the networks of service providers and consumers, and the organizations which structure their interaction.

The middle-sized circles represent the most important and immediate subsystems to be considered, that is, the specific organizations which the consultant and consultee represent. Finally, the immediate point of contact within these fields of influence are the consultant and consultee.

7. **That does not tell me what things I must understand in order to use the social systems context in consultation.**

Then let's look at what the elements are that one should have in mind and understand. To begin with, let us focus on the organization to which the consultant or the consultee belongs. An organization is a special entity with a name and place: for example, "Central Mental Health Center," or "Aaron Burr Junior High School." Here are six additional components found in any organization:

    A. *Goals and objectives:*

        1) There are stated goals: Where are they set down? (Code? Law? Policy? Constitution?) How is success in achieving the goals measured and by whom?

        2) There are also unstated goals: What do those working in the organization try to achieve that is not officially stated? Who decided these goals? The admini-

stration? The staff? Consumers? The legislature? A
board of directors?

For example, a clinic's stated goals are to provide
direct treatment to adults in the community. The
admission workers have agreed to take no new
chronic schizophrenic cases. This unstated goal
developed because they feared they would have to
close new admissions if their caseload became
jammed with chronic patients.

B. *Physical space:*

What is the real estate like? The buildings? The equipment? What does the consultant sense when he first sees
the physical space? (Understanding the physical space is
like understanding the nonverbal characteristics of a
patient: his gestures, facial expressions, etc.) What about
its size? Is it clean or dirty? What are the offices like?
Does it have a library and equipment to do the job?

What is the first thing the consultant is shown when
looking around? Why do they *wish* to show him that
first? What is shown first may indicate what the consultees value or what they think the consultant values.
Examples: In the old state hospital the floors were clean
and antiseptic but the patients were deprived of opportunity for self-expression. A littered, dirty office may,
however, suggest something about the lack of care among
those who work there.

C. *Organizational structure:*

What is the table of organizations? What are the roles?
What status is applied to various roles? What is the
hierarchy? What about budget and salaries? Is there an
informal structure?

Some index of the usefulness of the formal structure
can be obtained by gauging the strength of the informal
structure. If these structures are rigidly maintained and in
opposition, it suggests the failure of both. How rigidly are
the roles prescribed and limited, or how ill-defined and
loose are they? Does the administrator have greater status
than the highly skilled worker? Has the organization
enough people to carry on the administrative maintenance functions, or is it top-heavy? Is the budget
adequate and are salaries adequate to retain personnel?

D. *The people (personnel and client):*

Who are the people? What is their education? How are they recruited? How are they integrated into the system? How is the morale? What about the communication? Who talks to whom? How much turnover and mobility is there? Who are the first people who seek out the consultant? Are they "ins" or "outs"? To whom do you have access in the organization? To whom is access denied?

At the boundary are the organizational members who are most like the outside community and least like those responsible for the administration and maintenance of the organization. The members who are open to the entry of an outsider may not speak for the organization. They may actually be deviant members and, in the case of consultation, the ones most like the consultant. If the consultant wishes to have an impact on the whole system he must not too quickly align himself with those who reach out and accept him. He must realize that they are probably not representative of the whole organization.

E. *Stages of development:*

In some ways the developmental stages of an organization are like those of a person.

1) Infancy: Is the organization new? Have its organizational components been differentiated yet? Does it have a stable budget and a history of success, or is everything in the future?

2) Maturity: Is there justifiable satisfaction and pride in the organization? Are there adequate stable resources? Continuity in the staff and functions?

3) Senility: Has it lost touch with its tasks and the community? Has it become obsolete? Have the maintenance functions taken precedence over the service functions?

The infant organization may much more readily admit a consultant. If there is little or no resistance to the consultant's entry, it would suggest that the organization seems to have little to protect. If it is senile it may put every effort into resisting, clinging to its life. The mature organization has a reasonable resistance to any entry. It values what it has and wishes to keep it. It is secure enough to consider change without panic.

The stage of maturity has little or nothing to do with the age of the operation. Unlike human development, an organization need never become senile. It can continually adapt to changing forces.

F. *The community:*

Does the organization reflect the community in which it exists? Is it more closely related to some distant community? Is there community pride in the organization? Community involvement? Community disdain? Community fear? Or is there only community ignorance of the facility? A mental health center canvassed the surrounding community to determine attitudes and found that very few of the residents had ever heard of it or knew of its existence.

8. **What special things should a mental health consultant keep in mind about his own system?**

The mental health system forms a reference group and determines much about the attitudes of its members. These attitudes are accepted by nearly all of them and so may appear to them as universal truths. But actually, these views may not be the same as those held by one of the consultee's systems.

For example, in the clinical setting there is a shared concept of what a "good patient" is. He is a person who is sensitive and openly expressive, among other things. This is an ideal toward which therapists strive. It is appropriate, since many patients are constricted and overly controlled. Therapists often work towards overcoming the crippling effects of the overly disciplined personality.

In other systems such as welfare, probation, or education, a sense of discipline may be the ideal characteristic of the "good client" or "good pupil." Success in a probation case is to be able to "keep clean" and out of trouble; for the welfare recipient it is to be able to work effectively; and for the student it is to be able to use his learning skills. All of these are examples of *increased* self-discipline.

The mental health consultant must be aware that his view of clients is derived from the clinical setting. It is not necessarily appropriate to the purposes of the consultee agency. The consultant must be open to reviewing and understanding the goals and requirements of the consultee system. If he is to be useful he must be willing to consider what he knows in the light of these new and important elements.

The mental health consultant's view of behavior is from a psychopathological perspective. He must also keep in mind that the staffs, clients, and pupils of the consultee's system do not regard themselves as "sick." They have not identified themselves as patients and are not looking for treatment as such.

In the mental health program, concepts and expressions referring to psychopathology represent the working language. In a consultee system these same expressions may appear "loaded." They may be potentially offensive or destructive to the self-concepts of both providers and consumers of services in the consultee system and alien to the system's goals.

9. **Are there any general characteristics of consultee systems which need to be remembered?**

Most of the consultee systems, like the ones we have mentioned, are public services supported by tax money and have these characteristics:

A. The administrators and workers in the system are under constant pressure. The consumers demand more service and are becoming better organized to demand it. Taxpayers, on the other side, are becoming less tolerant of expenditures and less willing to provide support. Legislatures and other branches of government are "investigating" the "abuses" in the systems. All of these create pressure, instability and insecurity for those trying to provide services in these systems and may make it difficult to do a good job.

B. The systems are organized as bureaucracies. They are generally very large organizations established and organized by public codes, laws, and rules. They have elaborate hierarchies for control which tend to separate each level from the next and from sources of power. There is often, as a result, confusion between what is legally required and what has been developed as unwritten policy to stabilize the organization.

C.   The structure, as a result, seems rigid and those who are committed to it assume an understandably defensive posture. Effective change in the organization must not be so rapid that it increases the threat to an already threatened organization. Further threat further diminishes the effectiveness of workers.

While mental health consultation works for orderly and responsive change, it also acknowledges that the work of the organization must go on from day to day in order to serve the current consumers. This may be the greatest contribution a mental health consultant can make, for while others call for what the system should be like tomorrow, the mental health consultant helps those within the organization to deal with the problems of today.

D.   Staff mobility and turnover occur at a high rate in these systems at all levels. Sometimes administrator and staff are systematically moved from branch to branch of the same organization, causing further instability. These factors may tend to reduce job satisfaction, morale, and commitment, since the workers cannot rely on a stable group of people in the organization. "Why try to do a good job if you won't be here tomorrow?"

Here the mental health consultant has something important to offer, for he can help the workers keep the focus on the task at hand.

10. **How does all of this affect the reception the consultant receives?**

Such agencies and their workers are in great need and often eager for help, even though they do not know precisely what kind of help they can hope to get. The mental health consultant arrives as a highly paid public employee of high status. He comes from the system of public service which, so far, has received the least organized public pressure. Thus, the mental health consultant arrives with a charismatic aura. A hazard exists when the need for an omnipotent savior in the consultee agency is matched by the consultant's need to be omnipotent. Should the consultant try to live up to unrealistic expectations, he may find some short-term gratification but, in the long run, the consultation program is doomed. Here are some of the problems which can be created when the consultant is tempted to respond to the desire for an omnipotent savior and is seduced into doing his "own thing" without regard for the system.

A. An enclave of "believers" develops, aligned with the consultant but representing a foreign body in the organization.

B. Workers may become incapacitated as they try to live under conflicting directions. Their morale and effectiveness may become impaired.

C. The organization may get rid of the consultant. In the consultee facility, the mental health program and its consultation project may develop a "bad name." Many consultee organizations are strong enough to get rid of the consultant: consultees do not appear at scheduled times or they make poor use of the time and eventually the contract is either terminated or not renewed. Unfortunately this then deprives the organization of a potentially valuable preventive tool.

---

exercises for chapter 3

Work as individuals, or if there is more than one person from the same agency, work in teams.

1. Define the organization for which you work in terms of the six components described in the preceding text:
   A. Goals and objectives
   B. Physical space
   C. Organizational structure
   D. The people
   E. Stage of development
   F. The community

2. If you are working in teams you may find that each person may have a different view about a particular component. Discuss why these differences have occurred and how an individual's role in the organization may have determined his different perspective.

3. You may find that there are important pieces of information which you do not have. Consider why this is. Does it make your work easier in any way to not know? Does it make your work more difficult in any way? Are there any other effects?

4. You may have found that you have some information about the organization which you would rather not share with other members or outsiders. Who specifically would you not wish to have a piece of information? What would be the potentially hazardous effects?

5. Define an organization to which you are a consultant in terms of the components described above.

6. Identify the kinds of information which you do not have. Speculate on reasons why you do not have this information. Are there reasons the organization might prefer you not to know?

7. What are the staff expectations of clients coming to your mental health program? What are the concepts of "good" and "bad" clients?

8. What are the staff expectations of clients who come to the consultee organization? What are the concepts of "good" and "bad" clients?

9. Compare characteristics of the mental health program with those of one or more consultee agencies. Using the six component parts described above, note differences and similarities.

CHAPTER 4

The Interface Between Consultant and Consultee

1. **You have talked about the social system context of consultation. What about the consultant and the consultee?**

   Since we have defined the circumstances in which they generally meet, we can now discuss the consultant and consultee from the standpoint of their individual needs.

2. **Let us begin with the consultee's needs. I think I already know a considerable amount about my needs as a consultant.**

   Following is a list of some of the hopes and needs of a single consultee (or a group of consultees). Each need is reasonable but not necessarily within the capacity of the consultant to provide.

   A. He wants to *get rid* of a troublesome client by getting someone "more competent" to deal with the problem. In other words, he wants to pass the troublesome client on to you.

   B. If he cannot get rid of the troublesome client, he would like to get a curative "prescription" for him. In other words, he wants to learn some of those "magical secrets" that he assumes you, as a mental health professional, possess.

C. He may want you for purposes of legitimization. He wants your blessing. He may consider his own position, experience, and training inadequate, and thus may want you to anoint him as part of what he considers a more prestigious network—mental health.

D. He would like you to confirm his work and reassure him about his competence. You will recall that the consultant must be careful about judging the competence of the consultee, since that can only really be done by someone in his own network, such as his supervisor. Therefore, the consultant cannot really confirm or reassure him about his decisions or their results. The consultant can, however, confirm the healthy nature of the consultee's efforts in attempting to seek a solution.

E. He wants you as a power tool to "straighten things out" since he believes you are more powerful than he. He wants to use you or get you to change his superiors or, if he happens to be a supervisor, to change his subordinates. He wants your power as additional leverage in dealing with his clients or their parents, or perhaps in dealing with the pressure brought on him by the community.

F. He wants you as a comforter, counselor, or therapist. He wants you to make him feel better and to make him stronger. If the consultant is also a psychotherapist he has to be very careful about this. The consultee is likely to appear like one of those long-sought "good neurotics:" the ones who are most able to use his psychotherapeutic skills.

G. He really wants a parent. He would like to have a father to give him advice. He would like to have a mother to nurture and comfort him. He remembers the "good old days" when he didn't have to face the hard realities of work and he could rely on his parents to take over in difficult times.

H. He would like to have a mature, interdependent growth relationship with someone from a different field who brings different experiences and skills. He would like this to be a relationship of mutual respect and one in which he feels he can trust the other but has something important to offer himself. This is the need the consultant hopes to find and the one he will nurture. This is *not* to imply that the others are "bad," but this is the optimal relationship. However, it is an ideal which is never fully realized.

3. **I can see my work is cut out for me. Maybe I am not so sure as I thought about my own needs as a consultant. Can you tell me some things to look for?**

Let's look at it the same way we did for the consultee. What are the consultant's needs and hopes? You will begin to see some wide discrepancies between the needs of the consultant and those of the consultee. These require negotiation. The following is a list of some of the consultant's typical needs both conscious and unconscious.

A. He needs to keep the consultee's client from becoming identified as a patient, so that he can cut down referrals to the mental health clinic. The consultant has gone into the consultee agency in order to prevent mental and emotional disorders, and that means keeping people out of the psychiatric treatment network.

B. He needs to find a place in the community to land in keeping with his program's goals of community coverage. Some categorical funding sources require that staff time be spent doing consultation. The program administrator in the mental health center may say something such as: "Everyone should be doing some community consultation. If you are not, find yourself a consultation."

C. He needs to be an infiltrator, a saboteur, a motivator for the "good purpose" of bringing the people in this "inferior" consultee organization "up to his level." He assumes that since he is a consultant he should know how the consultee organization should function.

D. He wants a pupil to teach. He has subject matter he values from his training in the mental health field. He has always enjoyed being a teacher and the consultees look like a good student population; they are bright and eager, and seem to respect him.

E. He wants someone to dominate. He has never cared much

for administrative responsibilities but has a good idea how organizations should be run. In the consultee organization there may be a possibility of getting people to do the things he has always wanted to try without being accountable. They respect him and think he has "the answers."

F. He wants to get out of the office. He wants to get around and see things in the community and what is going on in other organizations. He considers this a part of his education.

G. He wants to get away from "ungrateful" patients who are constantly demanding more than he can provide in direct services. Patients do not always get well, no matter what you do, and it can become agonizing to have to face unresponsive cases.

H. He wants to get away from organizational in-fighting. The social systems issues where he works are oppressive and he wishes to go somewhere as an "honored guest," insulated from office politics.

I. He would like to increase his reputation and visibility. As a consultant he is likely to become better known; people can see how "really competent" he is. It may be a good way to build a private practice.

J. He would like an interdependent growth relationship with someone from another field with different experiences and different skills. He values his own competence but realizes its limitations. He would like it to be a relationship of mutual respect where he can trust the other and increase his own potential. In actual fact the consultant may be mature enough to view consultation this way but probably also has many of the other needs mentioned above. If he knows what kind of relationship he is seeking he is more likely to find it.

The other needs may seem like "bad" ones and this the only "good" one, but they are all common realities of professional activity. They must be acknowledged as such in order that the consultation can begin to move in the direction of the more ideal interdependent relationship.

4. I can see that there *are* some wide discrepancies between the

consultant's needs and the consultee's. I like that idea of the interdependent growth relationship. But how can you reach that point in light of all these other things?

The discrepancies need to be discussed and brought out into the open in both the contractual arrangements and the on-going relationship.

5. I'm not sure I would feel comfortable being frank about some of the things you've mentioned and some of the other feelings I might have about what I want or need from the consultee and his organization. In fact, I can see myself trying to suppress my concerns.

That, of course, is one of the fundamental issues between the consultant and the consultee. Each has a basic fear. The consultant's fear is that he will appear inadequate in the eyes of the consultee or perhaps in his own judgment. The consultee's fear is the same. This makes it difficult to be open.

6. How can the consultee respect me as a consultant if he knows these "inappropriate" needs that I have? Isn't it better to keep quiet about one's own problems?

I didn't mean to imply that the consultant should immediately reveal everything about himself. That could possibly discredit his position and turn it into a problem-solving relationship for him. If some of these things are important, however, the consultant needs to accept that and be aware that they are issues for him. To be a good consultant you need to be as accepting of your own needs as you want to be of the consultee's. If you try to deny them they are likely to interfere with what happens. As you know from your clinical training, suppressed needs are likely to appear in some disguised form and further complicate the consultation. How much you reveal is an issue which can be decided only in the context of what is happening. Most of us feel better when not too much is hidden, but the important thing for the consultant is to be constantly considering this question: What is the best relationship for him, or them, and me? In a larger sense the question is also, what is the best relationship between his program and mine? There is no infallible prescription for this, any more than for any problem a consultee presents. The question must be kept open.

7. **It almost sounds as if the consultant has no firm place to stand. That sounds very ambiguous.**

   In fact, I believe that is true. The position of the consultant is an ambiguous one. He is at the boundary of his own organization and at the boundary of another organization. We know from research studies that "boundary people" are the ones most apt to experience role conflict. Under conditions of role conflict it is very tempting to try to prematurely effect rigid closure in order to promote a feeling of greater security. However, the effective consultant must be willing and able to tolerate a high level of role ambiguity without providing an immediate solution.

   In a sense, he is always asking himself the following questions: Who am I working for? My program? His program? The consultee himself? The community? The answer to all of these is yes. At any one given time one of these answers may appear in the foreground. However, there is a constant fluctuation in needs, as discussed earlier.

8. **I am aware that, as a consultant, I thought I would be getting away from some of the organizational stresses at the mental health center — the "systems problems." However, if I try to avoid some of these complications, I can see that I might be a less effective consultant than if I were willing to accept them as problems.**

   Yes, mental health professionals are sometimes tempted to become consultants in organizations where they are not held accountable for results and can act without reference to their effect on the system.

   For the person considering doing consultation, the central question is: Is consulting for me, or do I prefer clinical work, or teaching, or research? These are all legitimate possibilities open to the mental health professional. It's well for him to keep in mind an important issue that all professionals need to consider — who they *should* work with, and who they really *want* to work with. In the larger sense, since most mental health consultants are the representatives of a community-supported program, there is the question of whether it is the best use of public funds for them to do this job, too.

9. **I can see that these are things that I must really think about. I**

think I know what some of the issues are. Are there other things that I should keep in mind about the consultant-consultee interface?

One other element is important. It has to do with the permanence of a consulting job. The definition of consultant is "an outside agent" and if one continues as a consultant over a very long period of time, the question should be at least opened as to whether or not he has not started to do a staff job. The consultant should keep these questions in mind: "How can I work myself out of a job?" "Do they really need me?" "How long should I be there?" "Can they do without me?" He should be aware of termination in the same sense that he would be in one of the other helping roles he has, such as in psychotherapy. The consultant should be aware of the ambiguity of his position, especially if he actually wants to continue in the job and likes some of the adulation that he receives.

---

exercises for chapter 4

1. Work together in groups of three to develop dialogue around the cases which will be described below. One person plays the consultant, the second plays the consultee, and the third is an observer. Take five minutes for each case. The consultant portrays his role, while the consultee elaborates on the case material listed below. The observer tries to assess the ways in which the activities of the consultant and consultee move the relationship toward or away from "the ideal" of the mature, interdependent, respectful growth relationship in which each person experiences himself as competent.

    Following the five-minute consultation, the observer briefly reports his observations to the others. Then all three take two minutes to discuss the experience.

    Then the three move on in rotation for the next case. For example, the consultant becomes the observer, the observer becomes the consultee, and the consultee becomes the consultant in the next consultation.

    Here are the cases:

A. A young social welfare worker asks to see the consultant. She tells him that she believes that one of her clients is "psychotic." She further says that she did not learn in school how to handle such problems. She asks the consultant to treat the patient on a visit to the agency.

B. A probation officer requests consultation. He says that he has a client in whom he has seen a "pattern." The man is an exhibitionist with a number of arrests. The probation officer says that he realizes now after getting to know the man that he exhibits himself immediately after he has a visit from his mother. However, he says, he cannot mention this to the client because the man is so fond of his mother. The probation officer says, "If you can just tell me what I ought to do, I think we could help this man."

C. You are a consultant to a church area including six different individual churches. Your contract has been made with the bishop and you visit individual ministers at their requests to consider problems. After several weeks at various churches you are called to a small central city church where there is a young minister. He tells you that he does not consider most of the activities of his church to be relevant to the needs of their parishioners. He says that he considers himself more "human-relations" oriented than theologically oriented. As an example of the needs, he tells you of a young couple who live with one set of parents and are having marriage trouble. He tells you that he has read a good deal about "family therapy" and would like you to supervise his work as a family therapist with this group.

D. A schoolteacher tells you of a young student who appears to him to be bright but has great difficulty in reading. He tells you that last week he told the parents of this child to get a private tutor for the child and to read to him at home for at least an hour a day. Anxious about what he has done, the teacher asks, "Did I do the right thing? I only want to help. I really need your opinion. Did I do the right thing?"

E. A social welfare worker tells you of a young man who has been on Aid to the Totally Disabled. Recently, a change in ruling eliminated this client from half of his current support. The social worker presents the case as one that should receive special consideration since the man has "suicidal potential." He makes a strong case for how a reduction in support might lead to a suicide attempt, and wants to know if you do not agree that it would be safer to keep him on the current level of support. You respond affirmatively in a tentative way, indicating that you would like to explore the situation more. The social worker seizes on the affirmative part of your statement and then goes on to say, "I am glad you agree with me because I have been having a terrible time with my supervisor. She says she thinks it's a bad idea to continue the level of support in this case. I appreciate your support." Continue the consultation from this point.

F. A young schoolteacher asks for an individual consultation session. He closes the door and says, "I realize that you're here as a consultant about the children but it's very clear to me that if I am to do a better job with them, what I really need is to work out a personal problem I have had for years. It has to do with my anger." He pauses a moment and then continues. "What I really mean to say is that I would like you to be my therapist when you come to the school each week."

2. Working in pairs, go back to the main part of the lesson and, individually, review the first nine of the needs listed for the consultant. Alternate the main responsibility for discussion of each item between the two of you. Take three minutes on each item. Consider that this particular need is a reasonable one for you to have as a consultant. Try to be as specific as possible how it relates to your own needs. What would be the effect of acting it out on a consultee and the consultee organization? Consider also how you might handle this need in such a way that it does not interfere greatly with your function as a consultant to the organization?

3. Now discuss the consultee's needs in the same way.

CHAPTER 5

The Entry Phase: Opening with the System

1. **Why do you call it the entry phase and make a special issue of it? Is there something different about its purpose?**

   The purpose of this phase is to develop, with the administrator's sanction, a contract or agreement about some joint work between the consultant and consultee.

2. **How do you go about it?**

   Much depends on how contact is made with the consultee system: whether they contact you or your mental health program for consultation, or whether you attempt to initiate a consultation program with the agency.

3. **Let's start with the easier situation.**

   That would be when you are invited by the consultee's system to be a mental health consultant.

4. **What should the potential consultant do at this point?**

   During the entry phase the consultant should perform the following activities in conjunction with the consultee system.

A. Explore the goals, objectives, and values of the potential consultee system in order to find some common base with the goals, objectives, and values of the mental health program. It is essential that both systems have some human values in common.

B. Explore the needs of the consultee system as the *administrator* of the system sees them.

C. Consider whether you as consultant have the specific expertise required by the consultee.

D. Develop agreement on the structure needed to carry out this consultation project. This structure includes specifics such as duration, time, place, and consultee groups or individuals needed to meet the goals. Such agreement requires coordination between the administrator's ideas of availability of space and personnel and the consultant's view of such matters as the effective size of groups, intervals of time, and duration.

E. Discuss the expectations of consultation. Specifically, this involves exploring the administrator's hopes and wishes and dealing with what may be unrealistic expectations. For example, sometimes an administrator will hope that the consultant will deal with a serious staff problem beyond the scope of the task identified for consultation.

F. Discuss the fee and how it is to be paid. There are several possibilities:
   1) A personal fee may be paid to the consultant.
   2) A fee may be paid to the consultant's system.
   3) There may be no fee. This is the most common situation for most public mental health programs.

G. Discuss ways of sustaining the consultation project. There are several specific issues in this sustaining process:
   1) The way in which the consultant will keep the administrator of the consultee system informed about consultation activities. It is well to describe what kinds of things will be reported and what kinds of things will be kept confidential. Trust within the consultee system requires open communication of all aspects of the system as well as confidentiality about individual persons active on any issues described.

2) The way in which the consultant can receive feedback on the impact of the project. Again, the issues of confidentiality and trust become important. There are certain kinds of things which the consultee may wish to share with the consultant but there are certain specifics which he may wish to keep confidential.

3) The importance of keeping communication open. This should be emphasized to the administrator.

4) A final report on the consultation project. This should be given to the administrator either orally or written. It is well for the consultation project to have some end in sight even if the contract is to be renewed. A report is generally given at the conclusion of a portion of the project or the total project.

H. Clarify to the consultee system that sanction on some of these agreements must be obtained from the consultant's system, and that the consultant will report their discussion to his own organization for further review. The issues chiefly requiring the support of the consultant's system are such specifics as time and duration. These are items that affect the consultant's system in its demands on his time and priorities. The consultant, however, should have autonomy in deciding with the administrator of the consultee system on other elements such as content and focus.

5. **Does the consultant discuss with the administrator the method of getting started with a group of consultees?**

It is important to discuss with the administrator the ways of introducing the consultation project into his system. This involves exploring the administrator's ideas and clarifying the importance of basic sanctions and clear methods of communication within the system.

6. **Is that, then, the end of the entry phase?**

Not quite. It's important to close the entry phase firmly and clearly. That involves two major procedures:

A. The mental health professional must notify the administrator of the consultee system that his own administrator has sanctioned the terms on which he is to become a consultant.

B. A formal or informal contract should be written, making explicit the terms of the agreement. This usually takes the form of a letter by the consultee agency's administrator. The consultant then confirms acceptance in a return letter. These letters do not have to be in formal "contract language."

7. **So much for getting administrative sanctions. Now, how do you begin consultation?**

The consultant has three main purposes in the opening phase of consultation.

A. To explore the *needs as the consultee sees them* in the context of the organization.

B. If personal needs and organizational restraints seem in conflict, to focus on the question of how the conflict can be resolved.

C. To make it clear that he, the consultant, is identified with the whole consultee system and its objectives, and to dispel any idea that he is there to either destroy or transform it. The consultant is employed to enhance the present system for more effective service.

8. **How are these objectives achieved?**

A. The consultant should make a simple statement about how and why he is there, acknowledging the legitimacy of the consultee's questions and his interest in exploring the consultation project.

The consultant should indicate that the important thing at the first session is to find things to work on together. He must try to steer clear of implying that consultation has been "ordered" by the administrator. If the consultees feel that the consultation project has been "ordered," the consultant may offer subjects for the consultees to consider for discussion.

B. The consultant should begin to explore the needs as the consultee sees them. He may wish to help group them into general categories, such as total system needs, organizational needs, program needs, community support needs, individual skill needs, etc. He should also try to name and set aside as inappropriate to this project any needs related to personal problems among personnel. However, it is wise to acknowledge any personal need expressed and see if it can be related in any aspect to an organizational or task issue suitable for discussion. In this process the consultant can clarify and relate himself to those needs expressed in the contract.

C. The consultant should state simply the agreements made with the system administrator. If little agreement on the needs can be seen between the administrator and the consultee, the consultant should express willingness to rediscuss the issue with the administrator.

D. He should state the agreements made regarding time, place, duration, etc. While not dwelling on the issue unnecessarily, he should invite the consultee's reactions and thoughts regarding commitment to the structural plan. He should be willing to rediscuss these structural issues with the administration if agreeable changes are suggested. If the consultees accept the consultation structure after suitable discussion, the consultant should not pursue differences, since the consultees may then feel that they "should" have differences and so may invent some.

9. **What you have been describing seems to be preliminary to the actual consultation process.**

In one way that is true, but it can also be viewed as an *integral part* of the process, as it provides opportunity for demonstration of the consultant's integrity, his initial identification with the consultee system, his sensitivity and thoughtfulness as a person, his openness to and acceptance of the consultee's reactions and ideas, his interest in a joint collaborative process, and his willingness to act as a link with other segments of the system when necessary.

10. **What are the next steps?**

They may be taken in the first session or in the second. They involve discussion and selection of content and ways of moving directly into consultation. This marks the end of the entry phase with the agency and the beginning of the consultative process with the specific consultees. The way of working most commonly suggested by the consultees is discussion of the case example.

11. **As you mentioned, these steps all follow when the consultant has been invited in by the administrator or consultee system. What happens when the consultant tries to initiate the consultation? That often happens in mental health programs.**

When the potential consultant initiates the encounter, the steps we have discussed may serve as a guide for an ideal transaction. But naturally there will be further problems in the transactions with the administrator and the consultee system.

12. **How does the mental health professional initiate a consultation?**

In formulating an approach, the consultant should keep in mind the following three factors.

   A. A sense of the common responsibility of the two service systems to the people of the community.

   B. A belief that, with common community objectives, collaborative efforts are more effective and economical than separate efforts.

   C. Recognition by the potential consultant that he is an intruder in the consultee system and so must be willing to absorb negative as well as positive emotional reactions to such intrusion.

13. **What if the mental health program administrator makes the initial contact with the consultee agency administrator?**

In that case the designated consultant need only confirm his understanding of the arrangements. In such relationships the flow of communication between the consultant and his own administrator is vital. Since additional levels of operation will be involved in both systems, the consultant must keep channels open. It may be that the consultant's administrator will maintain most or all of the contact with the consultee agency administrator. In that case, periodic reporting from the mental health consultant and administrator to the consultee agency administrator would be helpful.

14. **What if it is the mental health professional who makes the initial**

contact with the administrator of the agency where he seeks to be a consultant?

Sometimes this is a more difficult task, since administrators like to talk to administrators. But differences in size and prestige of programs may make it possible and effective. The consultant must be sensitive, however, to the significance of these status differences.

More often the consultant has access to an assistant administrator or training officer. In this case the potential consultant can work from preliminary discussions toward a meeting with the chief administrator. With such preliminary work done, discussion with the chief administrator can often be less detailed.

15. **What if the only access to the administrator of a potential consultee agency is through a supervisor or staff member — people more remote from consultee agency authority and decision-making?**

This, too, occurs often. After a preliminary discussion of the necessity for administrative sanction, you may be able to discuss with staff members and supervisors their willingness to take responsibility to work *within* the channels of the consultee agency toward the development of the project, and especially toward an eventual conference with the administrator or his delegated representative. Incidentally, it is worthwhile trying to make even brief contact with the administrator.

16. **Why do you emphasize contact with the administrator so much?**

If there is not at least visual contact between the administrator and the consultant the administrator may inadvertently or purposely remove sanctions, or the consultant may get caught in organizational in-fighting and unknowingly permit some misuse of his role and purpose. Contact with the administrator is one way of safeguarding the future of the consultation project as well as expanding the consultant's knowledge of the consultee system.

17. **Can you give us some tips about what to be aware of in contact with the administrator?**

Several major points should be emphasized.

A. The consultant should try to understand the reactions to his "interference" and also the fears and apprehensions related to mental health personnel in general and experts in particular.

B. The consultant should try to show his interest in all agencies in the area of his community mental health center, and to express his wish to know about the programs and services to community people. He may wish to emphasize the referral channels between the two agencies and the fact that he may be able to assist in this interface area. He can express his hope that the administrator will help him in his tentative plan: i.e., to start the visiting potential consultant on his quest for knowledge and understanding with the basic ground work in the consultee agency, and with the expectation that the administrator will turn him over to others for details.

18. **I suppose the ideal thing would be for the administrator to present his own administrative problem to the potential consultant.**

I think it might seem ideal at first. However, if that does occur, the potential consultant should acknowledge the problem as a worry and concern of the administrator; but I think it is better for the consultant not to offer help right then and there. He could say something like the following: "If it ever seems to you worthwhile to discuss a question such as that with an outsider, a staff member of our center is available. People have found that it sometimes helps them to straighten out the various parts of a complex problem; and *that* can lead to seeing more clearly what to do." In this way, the consultant will not jeopardize his position by starting to work on a problem before the ground rules have been laid. It may serve as an excellent opportunity to discuss the structure of a consultation project.

19. **There seems to be an ambiguous element in what you are saying. Although the consultant is there to help, you make it sound—in the case where the consultant tries to initiate the contact—as if he should be reluctant to start consultation. You also emphasized that the consultant should indicate what he would like to get from his contacts with the consultee agency, rather than what he can give. Isn't that just contrary to the "helping role" of the consultant?**

You may be forgetting that when the potential consultant initiates the contact, no one has asked him to help with anything. In my view, an honest stance for the potential consultant who initiates a contact is that he comes for something for himself and his mental health agency. If the potential consultant starts working on a problem (thus shifting his stance from seeker to helper) *before* the administrator hears about it and has a chance to help establish ground rules for consultative help, the risk of impulsive withdrawal is great. If the potential consultant maintains his original stance to find out about a particular community agency, he can gain information that will truly help him in his work.

If the administrator offers to discuss and show his agency in action, the potential consultant has taken a major step toward becoming a consultant to that agency. The would-be consultant in this case is visiting to ask a favor, not to offer good things.

20. But what if the administrator does not approve the request to learn about the organization?

If the administrator does not respond to the visitor's request, the visitor is held at this first barrier and should try to withdraw as gracefully as possible. He can say such things as, "I do realize you're very busy and I guess this was a bad time to put an extra demand on you and the agency," or "I should have waited until budget time was over." He may add, "When things lighten up a bit, I'd be glad to come over again."

21. How about the situation in which, after an initial rejection by an administrator, the consultant does get a contact with some other member of that agency?

The would-be consultant has no right to visit or "invade" other segments of the agency. If persons within the agency contact him he should redirect them to work through proper agency channels. Otherwise, as you can see, a situation could arise which would be very problematic for the future of consultation and for relationships with the mental health progam.

22. Does that mean, then, that if the first visit is not successful, the mental health professional should give up and wait to hear from the agency's administrator?

The would-be consultant should discuss the situation with his own director or other staff members to decide if work with the agency is important enough for a later effort. It may be that someone else in the mental health program could more effectively deal with the agency's administrator.

23. **Everything seems to hinge, then, on whether the administrator is willing to sanction the would-be consultant's entry, by either showing him the agency, telling him about the agency, or actually moving to request consultation help for his agency.**

Yes, that is true. It is not likely to be a simple yes-or-no situation. There are at least three major possibilities.

   A. The administrator may be warm, responsive, and seemingly eager to have the would-be consultant.
   B. He may agree grudgingly out of an inability to deny the request.
   C. He may agree in an ambivalent way, out of mixed feelings of warmth and pride about his organization and lingering fears and apprehensions about the intrusion.

The consultant should keep in mind that the quality of the administrator's sanction will affect the remainder of his reception and that there are "chain effects" to actions throughout the system. For example, the administrator's ambivalence may very likely be transmitted somehow to the other people the consultant will see. On the other hand, his warmth and good will could also be so transmitted. The communication may also have effects of another kind; that is, the administrator's reluctance to use the consultant may be at least in part dispelled by the reports he hears about how the consultant's contacts have gone.

24. **Well, that may mean that I should think more about the nature of those contacts.**

Yes, let me restate some of the points to keep in mind.

   A. Be sure to show appreciation and respect for what is given.
   B. Show regard for the time and effort of others.
   C. Make an effort to understand the long-term or short-term goals and objectives of the agency, and to demonstrate a grasp of the programs and services in the context of the agency's rules, structure, and procedures. To put it

another way, it is important for the consultant not to come with an obvious diagnostic stance, but to reveal himself as an appreciative visitor acknowledging the strengths of the structure and the tasks of the organization.

D. In the formal and informal encounters he has with people in the organization, it is very important for the consultant to demonstrate that it is a colleague relationship which he seeks. This is one in which he neither undervalues nor overvalues his role as a visitor, nor overvalues his role as a professional from another field.

E. Wherever possible, he should make an effort to be useful as he is being shown around. This does not mean that he should try to "sell his wares," but that he should contribute to the conversation. Where a question is raised, he should give freely of what he knows that is pertinent.

F. Another useful way of getting started is by agreeing to jointly examine some aspect of the collaboration between the potential consultee agency and the community mental health center. For example, the two might try to determine how many clients are being served jointly.

It is well to keep in mind that most people prefer to help rather than to be helped. This is especially true of people in the helping and service professions. The willingness of a potential consultant to ask for help, without compromising his confidence or his sense of competence, may be an important demonstration of a future model for consultation to the workers in the potential consultee agency.

---

exercises for chapter 5

Break up into groups of six. In each group, two people should work out an exercise, and the other four should help to evaluate.

In all the exercises, you are a staff member of a community mental health center.

1. A call comes to you from the director of the regional office of the county welfare agency. He has a communique from his central office stating that consultation is available from the local mental health center. He says, "My workers need all the help they can get, so when can you come over?"

   A. Pair off with another trainee who will take the part of the regional director.
   B. Play out this dialogue.
   C. The entire group of six should evaluate, question and discuss the dialogue.
   D. In light of the discussion, another pair should play out the dialogue. There should be no restraints on the requester of consultation.

2. A direct service staff member of the regional office of the county welfare agency calls you for consultation regarding a case in which she has much apprehension about the mental health of a mother. She asks, "Should I get her to a mental hospital?"

   Pick up the dialogue from here and follow the procedure in exercise 1.

3. The supervisor of a unit of six direct service workers and two aides calls you. She says, "At a community meeting I heard your name mentioned with high regard. My workers need to learn everything psychiatric. Could you give us some consultation? I'll set up a meeting." Enact this scene as in exercise 1.

4. A call comes to you from the guidance counselor of a nearby senior high school. She says she was intrigued by the newly painted name of the center, and a few days ago stopped in and picked up some brochures. She says, "Our school has plenty of problems. Right now our principal feels pushed about all the drop-outs. Would consultation cut down on the number of drop-outs?" Pick up the dialogue from here as in exercise 1.

5. A call comes from a teen-age boy who is a student at a nearby junior high school. He refuses to give his name, but goes on intensely and with much emotion to say, "It's about drugs. It's

awful! I know lots of guys who are strung out on them. I've had some, and I know it's not for me. Could you stop by the school yard and talk with some of the group? I wouldn't want them to know I called you." Enact this scene as in exercise 1.

6. Your director attended a community meeting where there was much discussion about drug use by teen-agers. The principal of the junior high school was present. On the whole, he appeared objective. His remarks were chiefly that drug use was pretty pervasive, and he didn't think much could be done about it. Your director asks you to visit the school to see if you can develop a consultation program with school staff. What would you do? Pick up the dialogue from here as in exercise 1, with another trainee taking the role of the school principal.

7. Four months ago when the center was newly opened, you wrote a letter to the principal of the nearby senior high school, setting forth the program and services of the new center and mentioning mental health consultation to schools as one of the center's special interests. You offered to discuss all this with him if he would set a time. You received no reply. Today the head counselor of that school telephones you, talks of the many problems of students in her school, and asks if they can have some consultation help for the teachers. You are responsive to her concern, but do ask if she has cleared with her principal about asking for some help from the center. She says, "No, I haven't. He is even more distraught than last term, and he has as much as he can do to keep up with all the projects that are now going on in our school. I thought I would save him adding another." Pick up the dialogue from here as in exercise 1.

8. Your director, in conference with the administrator of the local county welfare agency, gained sanction for a mental health consultation project for direct service workers and their supervisors. It was a superficial kind of sanction, with the local county welfare agency administrator saying, "Sure, come in and do what you can, but I'll have to ask you not to bother me with it, as I have ten other headaches that take priority over what my staff people don't know."

Under the leadership of an enthusiastic staff member, the

project got underway one and a half years ago and the consultant reported much initial interest and use by two supervisors and their twelve workers. The sessions focused on case consultation and discussion of workers' presentations. Interest dissipated during the year, however, and a number of times the supervisors said they needed to use the time for urgent agency business.

The first consultant has left the staff of the center and the director asks you to pick up his assignment. You go to the agency office a half hour earlier than the scheduled session time to introduce yourself to the supervisors. You are met in a business-like manner, far from inviting. After a few pleasantries, and much effort on your part to make some connection with the two supervisors, one of them blurts out, "Do we *have* to go on with this this year? What with the changes from Washington, and the Governor's cuts in budgets, we are just going from crisis to crisis." Pick up this three-person discussion and continue as in exercise 1.

CHAPTER 6

The Mental Health Consultation Process

1. **The last chapter dealt with the entry phase. What comes next?**

   I call it the mental health consultation process. Webster's Collegiate Dictionary defines "process" in two ways: "a phenomenon which shows continuous change over time," and "a series of actions or operations definitely conducing to an end."

2. **To what end? What is the objective of mental health consultation?**

   The objective is to help a consultee deal more effectively with some *particular problem* in his work. It is very important to keep that objective in focus, lest the consultation drift aimlessly.

3. **I notice that you emphasize *particular problem*. What different kinds of work problems are usually dealt with?**

   The particular problem might be in a case at the direct-service-to-client level. Another type of problem might be between a supervisor or administrator and an individual staff member. Another type of particular problem might be in the system of program delivery of service. Still another might concern how best to introduce and develop a new program. Another might involve an administrator's concern over some aspect of his role. For example, I recall a situation in which an administrator was concerned about his role with two deputy assistant administrators. The "particular problem" was confined to this circumscribed area.

4. **Do you think that mental health consultation can generally help a consultee to work more effectively with his particular problem?**

   Of course this depends upon the persons and circumstances of each consultation. I think the process is more effective when the consultee is free to accept, modify, or even reject any ideas that do not seem fitting or feasible to him in his agency function.

5. **The concept of the egalitarian relationship between consultant and consultee, and that of the freedom of the consultee to use or not use the counsel, are emphasized over and over again. Do you consider these to be *the* only delineation of mental health consultation?**

   Of course not. Members of the therapeutic professions are well aware of the many and varied approaches to people; and, as yet, we do not know enough about how change takes place to say that there is only one single approach.

   However, the model under discussion is one with which we have had a lot of experience, and which we value. Further, we believe that if someone knows one model, he can then develop his own variations on it depending upon his own experience. Without a model to serve as a structure for change, it is possible to flounder aimlessly.

6. **Let us be more specific. What are the functions of the consultant in the consultation process?**

   There are at least five.

   A. *To provide information:* material which is specifically pertinent to the consultee's dilemma. Perhaps the simplest example is that in which the consultee needs to know something about psychiatric treatment and how to get one of his clients into it. But of course the information can be any from the consultant's background which will help the consultee to deal with his problem.

B. *To help the consultee fulfill his own responsibility.* If, for example, the consultee's work responsibility is to assess financial need in order to distribute public funds for financial support, then the consultant tries to help him do this *without undermining the mental health of his client.* Perhaps a public welfare worker's distorted ideas about psychosis may be impelling him to push a plan for mental hospital care when it is not needed. A mental health worker would provide him with information to make a sensible decision. Also, the consultant should not encourage the consultee to undertake psychotherapy with his client, as that is *not* the function of his public welfare agency, and not part of the consultee's work responsibility.

C. *To keep the administration posted* (without violating confidentiality) on the course of the consultation program. We mention this again to emphasize the responsibility of the consultant to the system which he is serving.

D. *To collaborate with the consultee* at times by undertaking some action in the problem situation. For example, the consultee may wish the consultant to see one of his clients or pupils, perhaps in the classroom, or in a separate interview. The consultant may do so and then share his new information with the consultee. The consultant, of course, must guard against taking the case over from the consultee.

E. *To be a facilitator for or with the consultee* within the consultee's own system. There are many dangers in undertaking this last function: the focus must remain on the specific task, and respect for the competence and integrity of the consultees and system must be shown. The following is an example of such facilitation.

A group of social workers might suggest in a case-centered consultation a different way of doing intake which would speed up service to clients. In many instances, the workers could discuss their suggestions directly with their supervisors, but in some situations the consultant could be a facilitator between the group and the supervisor in arranging a hearing for the idea and in helping group members to understand any difficulties which the supervisor might envision in making a change. Functions A, B, and C are components of every consultation process. Functions D and E are performed only when they further the objectives of the systems of the consultant and the consultee and their joint program of consultation.

7. **I remember your saying that the consultant is responsible for the process of consultation, and that the consultee is responsible for any decisions or actions which come out of it. Does this suggest that the direction of the consultation is entirely in the hands of the consultant?**

No, I did not intend that inference, although I can see how you drew it. The consultant is responsible for some inputs and the consultee is responsible for others. The consultant, however, is the one to guide the consultation process and to organize it in time. The consultee's concern, of course, is with the outcome. The consultant must keep his eye on the objectives of the consultation process so as to help the consultee into a more effective stance in his own work and responsibility. There is a parallel between the form of this movement and that known in other therapeutic processes. The form contains a beginning, a middle and an ending, each related to a specific purpose in mental health consultation.

8. **What is first?**

In the beginning phase of the interaction process, the following considerations should be kept in mind.

A.   The consultant should be sensitive to any initial stress in the consultee and aware of his *own* stress also, if by chance it is present.

B.   The consultant should encourage the consultee to present his problem situation. If a written report has been submitted, the consultant may ask for a brief oral summary of the highlights.

9. **Why bother with an oral summary if a report has been submitted?**

An oral summary offers the consultee an early opportunity to talk about and elaborate something that he knows better than the consultant. If it is a long-term case or long-standing dilemma, the review may reinforce the consultee's impulse to get help with it. The summary also offers the consultant an opportunity to grasp the outline and details *as the consultee sees them* and to assess his understanding of both the whole and the salient details. If the consultee does not present a question or topic for discussion, a short oral summary is also a good device with which to begin the consultation.

10. **What comes next?**

The consultant learns more about the consultee and his situation through inquiry for detail and through exploration of areas which the consultant considers pertinent. This also sharpens the consultee's focus on the case and may reveal to him some meaningful areas for study.

11. **What is the consultant hoping to do at this point?**

Two things.

A. To grasp the details regarding the interaction between the consultee and the other people involved.

B. To understand the consultee's dilemma over his situation. For example: Is the consultee fearful of activity that will push his emotionally disturbed client into a psychotic episode? Is he apprehensive that explanation to his client of some agency limitation may bring forth more hostility than he can cope with? Is he fearful of his supervisor's disapproval? Perhaps he feels that a client who is neglecting her children should have them taken from her, but he is also aware that there are insufficient hard data for a court to accept such a plan. Perhaps the father in his client family reminds the consultee of his own, so that he feels uneasy and inadequate whenever the father is present at the interview. Perhaps the case is so heavy with interrelated problems that the consultee does not know where to begin.

12. **Much of the consultation for mental health programs is done with *groups* of consultees. Are there special procedures to be used with groups?**

The consultant should invite the participation of all the members in consultation. He may ask if they have any specific questions on the case situation, and if they have been in situations with similar concerns. When questions and topics for discussion have been offered by the presenter the consultant may ask if anyone would like to add others.

If the person who presents the problem situation carries the whole responsibility and the other members do not become actively involved, the session is likely to be a consultative process for the presenter and an educational process for the other members. That is, for the other members it will seem more theoretical.

13. **Getting started is one of the hardest things for me as a consultant, so I want to understand this beginning phase as fully as I can.**

The beginning stage *is* critical to the consultation process, because it sets the stage for what follows. Think of it this way:

    A. The consultant demonstrates both his interest in the consultee's situation and his dynamic involvement with the consultee in studying and thinking about it. A noncommittal "yes" in pauses, or a nod, does not generally express sufficient consultant involvement. It usually takes more feedback than that for the consultee or the group to sense the consultant's involvement.

    B. When working with a group, the consultant invites the participation of the others and works toward discovering the group's feelings. At the same time the consultant wants to maintain the focus of this feeling on the case under consideration, and not let it spread to personalities or unrelated issues.

    C. The consultant tries to be alert to early signs of group identification with or against the presenter or himself. He should try to be aware of any divisive elements which may be developing in the group.

14. **What pitfalls does the consultant face in this opening stage?**

    A. Getting caught in an exploration of intrasystem problems as the primary focus.

    B. Getting involved in the exploration of the personality problems of the consultee.

    C. Subtly transmitting the feeling that the consultee is incompetent. We have already discussed how important this issue is.

    D. Subtle and perhaps unconscious acceptance by the

consultant of the consultee's feeling that the consultant should assume responsibility for dealing with the problem presented. Sometimes it is as though an unspoken agreement has been entered into, and too late the consultant becomes aware that the whole problem has been dumped in his lap.

E. Exploration of the consultee's case situation in such detail that too little time is left to help with the dilemma itself or to close the consultation. The consultant must be aware of and responsible for guiding the *total process* of the consultation in the available time.

15. **Suppose that the consultant has survived the beginning phase of the consultation process. What comes next?**

The middle or sustaining phase of the consultation process. Let us consider it from the standpoint of what the consultant and consultee put into it. In a constructive consultation process, of course, the interaction of thought and feeling among the presenter, group members, and consultant is so constant that it is difficult to separate the inputs of each even for purposes of study.

The responsibilities of the consultant are to keep certain points in focus and to help the presenter and the group to move smoothly from one focus to another. The following is a useful sequence of focuses.

A. Diagnostic assessment of the case situation. For his own purposes and to help the presenter, the consultant will wish to assess the presenter's dilemma. Sometimes this is known and acknowledged by the consultee, sometimes not.

B. Exploration of possible approaches to the problem situation with the presenter and group members.

C. Active involvement in eliciting the reactions of presenter and group members to the various ideas and suggestions for action.

D. Keeping open the various suggestions so as to preclude premature closure. A single consultee, or a group, is sometimes eager to seize upon the first suggestion in order to demonstrate responsiveness and openness.

E. Focusing on the presenter's right and responsibility to select what procedures seem feasible for him. With the consultant's help, the presenter consultee usually is able to choose a direction for his activity that feels right in his problem situation.

16. **What pitfalls can occur in the middle phase of the consultation process?**

   A. The consultant may become involved in the consultee's personal problems. These tend to show up most often in the middle phase.

   B. Even though the consultant may not get involved in these personal problems, he may be so conscious of them as to lose sight of the consultee's strength and competence as a worker.

   C. The consultant may subtly or unconsciously assume some responsibility to "treat" the consultee, seeing him in the patient role.

   D. The consultant may lose track of time and not focus quickly enough on helping the consultee toward making *some* decision.

   E. The consultant may have a specific decision in mind which is subtly transmitted through emphasis, tone, and attention, so as to block the consultee's own choice. Whatever emerges from the consultation must "feel right" to the consultee, in the sense that he can see himself moving in the chosen direction.

   F. The consultee may directly, indirectly, or even unconsciously try to shift the decision to the consultant, rationalizing his need to do so. This is not a pitfall unless the consultant actually makes the decision.

17. **You have often spoken about a *decision* in the case, as though some kind of incisive action *should* be forthcoming. Is that what you mean?**

   Yes and no. A number of alternative results may come out of the consultation.

   A. There may be a decision that more information must be obtained from the client or the consultee's agency.

   B. There may be a decision to postpone action in the case until an additional agency decision is obtained.

   C. There may be a decision to handle the case by working

for a special exception to normal policy within the client agency.

D. There may be a decision for the consultee to work in a specific new direction with his client without a reversal of general policy.

E. There may be a decision for more study and another consultation before any planned action is taken.

18. That should bring us to the closing phase.

Yes; in each consultation there is a beginning, middle and end.

19. How do you look at the closing phase and its tasks?

I consider it from the standpoint of the responsibilities of the consultant and the consultee.

A. The consultee's responsibility is to share his questions and any uneasiness about moving ahead in the direction he has selected. If the consultation process has been helpful up to this point, most consultees can do this naturally and easily.

B. The consultant also focuses on the consultee's uneasiness and questions. Together they look for some way of dealing with them. Through sympathetic discussion of questions or doubts, the consultee may gain enough conviction and confidence to deal more effectively with his problem.

C. The consultant should be aware of cues from the consultee regarding his interest in further conferences. In doing this he must maintain his consultation stance and avoid eliciting "reports" in a supervisorial manner. Both the consultant and consultee can easily fall into this kind of quasisupervisorial relationship, which may limit the professional growth potential of the consultation.

20. Does that mean that the consultant is not permitted any expression of interest or care about what will happen? It bothers me to think the consultant might have to restrain himself from expressing what to me seems a natural interest in the results.

Yes, that is a very good point. A natural expression of interest should not be restrained, but the consultant should keep in mind that his activities must not interfere with the consultee's sense of competence and freedom in carrying on his work. The interest expressed by the consultant, then, should not be in the form of a firm expectation or demand.

Often the setting in which the inquiry of interest is made can help in reducing its "accountability" qualities. For example, in informal settings such as a coffee break, lunch, or chance meeting, or at the beginning of a consultation session when other members are gathering, such comments have less chance of conveying an inference that the consultant has misgivings about the consultee's competence.

21. **It seems to me, however, that evaluation is such an important part of our activity as mental health professionals that more opportunity for it should be built into the consultation model.**

Yes, I do agree with you. I believe, however, that it is important for the consultant to maintain a role allowing discussion of material which would be precluded by the constraints of performance evaluation. It is often useful to set up sessions specifically for review and evaluation of consultation *as an agency program.* Such sessions, however, should not be focused on any specific case or problem but on the usefulness to the consultees of the consultation project itself.

22. **We have talked about pitfalls that may occur in the beginning and middle phases of the consultation process. What are the pitfalls in the closing phase?**

   A. If the consultant does not allow enough time for the closing, the process may not come to a full and natural end. The consultee then is forced to leave with many problems explored .but few decisions made that could help him toward more effective work.

   B. Because of its personal satisfactions, the consultant or the consultee may prolong the consultation beyond the time when it is actually productive in solving a problem.

   C. The consultant may tend to slip into the role of a supervisor, appearing to evaluate and direct the consultee's work and to hold the consultee accountable to him for his performance.

23. You have stressed the importance of keeping the administration posted on what goes on in consultation. I realize this and yet I am also concerned about your other statement that the consultant must be very careful not to elicit or give "reports" on individuals in the consultee organization. Can you give me some guidelines about keeping the administration posted and keeping out of this reporting context?

    A. Establish in negotiation with the administration some form for two-way communication. The consultant should be responsible for keeping the administrator posted about the program, and the administrator should be responsible for sharing some feedback with the consultant. They should spend some time together for evaluation.

    B. Despite the reporting, the consultant must maintain the confidentiality of his work with individual consultees, the administrator, and other staff members. This means that he can report generalities about what is going on, so long as he does not discuss individual staff members or specific groups in ways in which individual members may be identified.

    C. The consultant should be clear about what kinds of information he will share. It is often a good idea to let the consultees, the administrator, and others know just what information will be passed on.

    D. The consultant should be honest in his evaluation of the consultation project. Most administrators want to know from both the consultant and consultees if the time allotted is being used to real advantage in helping to fulfill the basic objectives of the agency.

        To an early inquiry of an administrator, a consultant might say: "I think we've made a good start," or "I think we're having a slow start." At some later point when there may appear to be less resistance, the consultant might say, "I think we're moving right along. More people are getting into it now." And then, at a still later time, he could say, "You might think of some ways to get staff reactions about the consultation from within the agency. I would certainly be interested in what comes out of that. I'll be getting some reactions from them, too, but they might say different things within the agency than they say to me. We could discuss the two kinds of evaluations the next time we meet." In general, most administrators want to know the consultant's opinion on how the project is progressing. Most administrators do not want to be burdened with details.

24. In your effort to describe a cohesive process, sometimes I felt a little lost. Let me see if I can set this for myself. There's a beginning, middle and closing phase with the consultee system, i.e., the negotiations with the administrator of the consultee agency. There's a beginning, middle and closing phase with a group of consultees or with an individual consultee. There is a beginning, middle and closing phase even for an individual consultation session. Did I get what you mean?

Yes, and I appreciate your summarizing it so explicitly.

25. You have spoken of the ways in which the consultant can relate to the whole agency system and its subsystems as he deals with various groups of consultees. That implies some movement through the system from one consultee group to another. Can you elaborate on this?

Yes, I can describe one way, perhaps the most common way, in which this movement occurs. Please understand, however, that these things are determined by the point of entry, the nature of the system, and the needs of the consultees, as well as the consultant's skill and his own needs. The first group of consultees may well be the direct service staff, and the subject focus is often on helping them with cases. As they begin to see the benefits, their supervisors may then wish to have some consultation themselves, either separately or as part of the original consultation group. As the consultant's work in the agency progresses, and as he develops more understanding of the workings of the whole system, a middle-management group or an administrative group may wish to meet with him on a program question. You can see that, if the consultant has acted as a useful and responsible professional who knows his role and respects confidentiality, his contacts with various members of the system may eventually result in his being a direct consultant to the whole system.

exercises for chapter 6

1. You are a staff member of a community mental health center. You are consulting with the twelve teachers of the first three grades of an elementary school. You and your director have made the agreement with the principal, who is eager to have such help. The principal had planned to have a short meeting with those twelve teachers after her faculty meeting so that they would be ready for your first session the following Thursday. When you arrive, however, the principal explains that a school emergency had arisen which lengthened the faculty meeting, and in the confusion she forgot the plan to meet those teachers. She says: "I'll take you down and you can explain it."

   A. Divide into pairs, one person taking the part of the principal, the other person the consultant, and continue the dialogue.

   B. As a group, enact the consultation session, each member taking the role of consultant, principal, or a teacher. Enact a five-to-ten minute session with the principal present throughout and then with the principal introducing you and leaving.

2. Your director has made an agreement with a school principal for consultation with the ten teachers of his fourth, fifth, and sixth grades. You have had a good first session, mentioning the agreements and the interest of the principal and your center, and discussing a plan of consultation on problem cases. They seem responsive and interested.

   This is your second session. After a bit of social conversation, you ask: "Who has a case to present?" There is silence, and then some embarrassed laughter and a few faces turning impassive.

   A. Be the consultant, with ten other members as the teachers, for five to ten minutes. Continue the session.

   B. Reenact the consultation with a new consultant.

3. This is the third session with the group in exercise 2. The group does get going with discussion of a very aggressive, boisterous,

angry boy of twelve who has been a problem to nearly every teacher in the group. The young sixth-grade teacher who describes his behavior, with sympathetic testimony from the others, ends with: "I breathe a sigh of relief when he doesn't show up." The others laugh in sympathy, and she adds: "Maybe I feel I have a reprieve for a day."

    A. Be the consultant in this situation for five to ten minutes. Continue with the group session.

    B. Reenact the scene with another member as consultant.

4. Same case as in exercise 3. After some discussion with the group, an older teacher who has not spoken up before says: "I know Jimmie, too! I think you should pray for more days of absence and hope you can stick it out till he goes to junior high."

    A. As the consultant, try to deal with this situation for three to five minutes.

    B. Reenact the scene with another member as consultant.

5. You are a staff member of a community mental health center and are in the third session of a planned twelve sessions of consultation on client cases with a group of twelve direct service social workers and their two supervisors in the local district office of the County Welfare Department. You and your group have made a good start. This third session marks the second presentation of a case by a group member. She is very much involved in a large client family, knows a great deal about the family, and is eager to share all she has learned about them over the preceding two years. She is so much involved in talking about them that she is unaware that you have glanced at your watch several times, as more than half the allotted hour has been used.

    A. Be the consultant, with another member taking the part of the presenter, and try to intervene for a more effective use of time. Continue the session.

    B. Reenact the scene, with the presenter and consultant exchanging roles.

6. The director of your community mental health center has developed a group consultation program with the administrator of the County Welfare Department. It has been in operation for three years. One other member of your staff is already involved in

the joint program and you are asked to help because of the demand for more groups. You have made a good start with a group made up of twelve direct service workers and their two supervisors. This is your fifth of twelve planned sessions. At a slow point in what you feel is only a moderately productive case discussion, one worker says explosively: "I don't have any problems with my cases. I have problems with those clerks who can never find anything when you need it, and bring it to you two days late! I wish we could have sensitivity training, or something. Or maybe *they* need the mental health consultation!"

    A. Be the consultant for five to ten minutes, trying to deal with this explosive remark.

    B. Reenact the scene with another member of the group as consultant.

7. The director of a private adoption agency telephones the director of your community mental health center to say that he has an agency problem that he would like to talk over with "someone who knows mental health." Your director asks you to explore this. In summary, the adoption agency director describes the situation thus: The last two years have shown great decrease in numbers of babies free for adoption, in large part because of birth control and legal abortion practices. The agency now has more staff members than the volume of work demands. Its staff is professional (most with an MSW degree) and highly sophisticated. The director hates to let workers go. He says he understands there are great needs in the mental health area and he would like some suggestions of what kind of program to develop with some of his staff—a program of service that is really needed today.

    A. Divide up into groups of four, with two taking the parts of consultant and director of the adoption agency and the other two as observer-reactors. Continue the dialogue.

    B. Repeat, with the observer-reactors in the consultant and director roles.

    C. As the staff member of the community mental health center who went to explore the situation with the adoption agency director, present your exploration in *your center's* next staff meeting. Take ten to fifteen minutes presenting the facts of your exploration, and leading discussion on this community request for help.

Other members of the trainee group make up the mental health center's staff group of ten.

8. A Big Brother Association has developed a counseling service for teen-age boys who have problems in adjustment. The agency's counselors have made very good use of mental health consultation from your center for the past four years. You are very familiar with the agency through your steady work with staff members and with the director for two of those four years. You are in the midst of a planned series of ten consultation sessions, which are going quite well. In this seventh session, a young man who has presented several cases over the years is especially angry over a policeman's arresting one of his boys for violating curfew. The man feels that the boy's arrest grew out of his defiance and assertions against the policeman rather than the violation of curfew rule. The man is not only angry with the officer but very admiring of the boy's behavior. He says, "You *got* to defend yourself in this world, and Jim had real guts! I wish I'd done that to my father long ago. I'd be better off than I am now."

    A. Be the consultant with that group of ten boys' counselors, and try to meet this situation. Ten other members should take the parts of agency counselors, and one should play the case presenter. Continue the session.

    B. Imagine this same incident occurring in an individual consultation session. Divide into groups of twos. Each group should enact a ten-minute consultation and then reenact it with changed roles.

9. The director of a district office of public health nurses sponsored a mental health consultation program with your center. You have carried on a planned series of twelve sessions which you and the nurses think have been helpful and effective. The sessions have become very relaxed and enjoyable. In the eleventh session, one nurse says: "Do we *have* to stop next time? I don't see why, when the sessions are so helpful." Others chime in and the good feeling seems pretty general.

    Be the consultant with this group of fifteen public health nurses for five to ten minutes. Continue the session.

10. A social worker, with over fifteen years of successful experience in community organization work, has developed against great odds a program called "Hot Meals for the Elderly." It grew out of a request to her from a neighborhood church that wanted "to do something to help our aging members." Many of the people were homebound, lived alone, and could not get to church. Starting with this one church, the social worker got this program going with the aid of volunteers and the church's advisory board. By dint of untiring work, two trips to Washington, and laboring over requests for grants, she got a grant for three years to enlarge the program and get it on a solid footing. This was a big and demanding community organization job. In the middle of the third year she was notified the grant would not be renewed because of across-the-board budget cuts, and "because this is such a small operation." The social worker has put "heart and soul," as she says, into developing this much-needed program of service. She is in a frenzy of activity to prove the need for this service. The social worker phones you at your community mental health center, as you have been on a community committee together, and asks you to help her support this program from the point of view of the mental health needs of elderly people, and to write a letter on the mental health hazards if the program is discontinued.

Divide into pairs and continue this dialogue for about ten minutes.

CHAPTER 7

Generic Elements
of the Consultation Process

1. We have spent a considerable time talking about establishing the structure of consultation, getting started, and keeping the process going. Yet what am I actually doing as a consultant to help?

   I am sure you were faced with this same question when you were beginning your clinical training, say, in psychotherapy or casework. What the consultant brings, mainly, is himself; he lends himself in a nondemanding, confidential, and trusting way to someone struggling with a problem. In the case of consultation, we have emphasized the system and structural elements so that, in addition to lending himself, the consultant can help to keep the focus clear. He may also sharpen the focus by commenting on or raising questions about certain structural elements which he can see as influencing factors.

2. What actually happens that is useful to the consultee? To use your metaphor, what is the content within focus?

   I can best discuss this by describing what happens to provide help in the consultation process: the generic elements of the consultation process.

3. What are these generic elements?

The first point I would like to talk about is very much like the placebo effect in medicine. In that case a person is in need, and what the placebo does is to introduce something new into the situation. We know from studies in both medicine and psychology that a new element may change the balance even though the new element may be a rather inactive one. When the consultant comes to meet with the consultee there is an implicit assumption that he can help. His status, prestige, interest and concern all come to bear on the problem. The consultee is aware that something new has been added, even before consultation. That something new is the hope that things can be better.

It is very important for the consultant not to minimize this effect. If he does he may undermine its usefulness. Let me give an example that I have encountered a number of times. A consultee requests some mental health consultation. He has a very troublesome problem, perhaps even a crisis. However, the consultation does not actually take place until several days later. When the consultant finally arrives, the consultee tells him that things are better, that the client has settled down, and that it does not seem as much of a problem as it was.

What may have happened here is that, in anticipation of the consultation, the consultee has begun to focus in a new way on the case. A new ingredient has been introduced. The consultant has been used though he has not yet appeared. However, without the consultant's agreement to help no change would have occurred. The consultee has used the consultant in fantasy, examining the case from this new perspective. The consultant's willingness to help has given the consultee a new ingredient and allowed him to make some major and important adjustments.

It is important for the consultant not to minimize or undermine this kind of reaction, or to feel hurt because the consultee seems to have worked things out alone. He has, in fact, given something very valuable by his willingness to lend himself to the situation. This is one of those situations where the consultant can, by his emphasis on the competence and capacity of the consultee, confirm what has gone on and aid materially in the case.

4. I would have thought of that as being simply a side effect. I can

see, though, that it is possible to enhance this "placebo" effect or undermine it by one's attitude. What is the next nonspecific element?

The next one is related but somewhat different. The consultant should try to view the consultee-client interaction as an unique human experience with growth potential in it for both. If the consultant conveys that he sees value in the consultee-client relationship, the consultee may begin to think of the client as more than just a painful irritant that he would like to get rid of—so often the way human services workers view troublesome clients. If, in working with the consultant, the consultee can gain in his own sense of competence, he may look upon this client experience as something to seek rather than to avoid. With the help of the consultant, the consultee can begin to see the growth potential for him in his work with the client; it becomes a challenging opportunity.

5. That is very interesting. I think I have had that kind of experience in getting consultation about psychotherapy and I can recall what a difference it made in my attitude toward seeing a patient. What is next?

Usually when the consultee brings a case to a consultant, he has reached the end of his rope. He would like to get the whole thing over with somehow. His ability to be a "helper" has been curtailed by a stubborn client who refuses to be "helped." The consultee then may look to the consultant for what can be called "the instant final solution."

Now, what the consultant can bring to this is an attitude which will move the consultee from his quest for an "instant final solution" toward seeing the client's troublesome behavior not as something that interferes with his job but as *part* of his job.

In one sense what happens is that the consultant accepts the consultee's dilemma but offers an alternative way of working on it. He implicitly conveys his view that the problem will not be solved instantly but only as an interesting *process* that has emerged in the consultee's work. This tends to counteract the despair the consultee feels and his desire to get the problem "over with." The effect of this loss of despair can in turn be very important to the client.

6. **Is there a generic element, as you call it, that can help me to think about the kinds of things I would actually say to a consultee?**

Yes. We are concerned with developing a more competent consultee. The kinds of statements which I believe are likely to promote this effect are those which recognize and acknowledge the healthy striving of the consultee to do his job. We spoke earlier of how a clinician must begin to think a little differently when doing mental health consultation. He needs to think in terms of the *strengths* he can see in the situation and to focus on those to a greater extent than he might in a pathologically oriented clinical stance. This means accepting the consultee, respecting him, and assuming that he is trying to do the best possible job.

Let me give you an example. A probation officer tells you, as a consultant, about his rage toward a client. He berates this client for not adhering to the probation rules. It would be tempting for a clinician to pick up on the rage as a personal characteristic of the probation officer with something like, "I can see how furious you are. Do you often have this kind of feeling?" This kind of statement may be appropriate to psychotherapy, in which the person has presented himself as the problem. However, in con-sultation you should seek the role-related aspects of the activity when making your comments. More than that, if you can find some aspect of it that seems indicative of a healthy role-striving, you should focus on that. For example, you may say, if you can see some evidence that this is the case, "I can see how frustrating it must be for you in your work with this man when you want so much for him to succeed in his probation."

7. **I can see the difference but it strikes me as being somehow dishonest or just playing with words.**

Of course, if it were really a dishonest statement, you would not want to make it. However, the awkwardness may only signify that the focus is different. You must decide for yourself. To be sincere and honest is more important than any technique. As a clinician you have no doubt developed a particular slant on things, a group of concepts that focus in a particular way, and it may feel a little out of place to begin to make observations and comments in other terms. I hope, though, you can see that this kind of comment is more likely to leave the consultee at the end of the consultation more able to do his job and with a stronger sense that he is a competent person. If the consultee can see his job with a particular client, and perhaps with most of his clients, as something worthwhile and a valuable continuing process, he will probably do a better job.

8. **I am aware that I have a tendency, developed in my clinical training, to view interactions, even in social situations, from the standpoint of the psychopathology that emerges. Are there other things that will help me in thinking of the kind of comments that I might make?**

A lot of what goes on in the mental health consultation process falls within what I call the "definitional process." In this process the consultant asks questions about the consultee's role with a specific client and how it relates to other situations. He wants to know as much as he can about the perspective in which the consultee views the situation. This is done with questions about the usual mode of operation in similar cases, the availability of resources, the circumstances under which the client is seen, etc. In this definitional process the consultant will express the things occurring to him that relate to his own role—ways in which his own work with clients is similar and ways in which it is quite different. He should do this not to imply that the consultee should imitate him but simply to define the similarities and differences in their roles. It is a differentiation process. The consultant wants to be sure that the organizational functions and constraints are defined in the situation as a part of the process: the roles of the supervisor and the administrator, and the laws, rules, or codes which determine certain operations. This will often bring to light structural or personal resources which, for one reason or another, the consultee has overlooked. It will also help the consultee to keep the focus on his work and the task to be done.

9. **Earlier you spoke of reverberations through the system. That seems rather vague to me. Is there some conceptual way of looking at that?**

Yes. A very neat scheme was developed from a slightly different vantage point. It's called the *parallel process* and is visualized in the form of a rhombus:

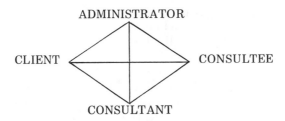

You will notice that at the four corners of the rhombus there are the administrator, the client, the staff member and the consultant. Each of these individuals has contact with the others, forming a number of dyads. The basic concept is that what happens in any one of these dyads is likely to be reflected in the others. This is understandable because there is an overlap of the individuals involved and they work toward the same end.

For an oversimplified example, let me begin with a situation not including the consultant. Consider, for example, an organization in which the administrator is very authoritarian and staff members are very obedient. One would expect to see this reflected in the relationship between staff and client as well. Probably staff members would reflect an authoritarian attitude toward clients, who would be expected to be obedient.

In an opposite view, if clients of an agency often present themselves as inadequate, incompetent people, the staff members may then see themselves as inadequate in their helping tasks. This, in turn, may produce a sense of great inadequacy in the administration. On the other hand, a marked division between attitudes of inadequacy and supercompetence may appear in dyads. The stance of incompetence in a person in one of the dyads is compensated for by a stance of supercompetence in the other: an administrator, for example, is viewed as competent but with an incompetent staff. Staff members are viewed as competent and clients as incompetent.

Another example of this kind of attitude reflection is seen when there is a hostile, aggressive stance by staff and a passive aggressive stance in clients or administration. In neighboring dyads, one would see a split between hostile-aggressive and passive-aggressive in some way. One can theorize which kind of split might occur in various organizations (probation, welfare, schools, etc.), depending on the client-staff-administration relationships.

10. **Where does the consultant come into this?**

The consultant affects the rhombus just as the others; in fact, that is a major point of leverage for consultation. Consider, for example, what can happen when the consultant enters an organization where people are divided by issues of adequacy and inadequacy. A worker presents a case showing how incompetent he is with a client. It may be tempting for the consultant to present himself as an all-knowing person, since he can give advice and not be accountable. If the case goes badly it will only confirm the consultee's incompetence. Reflections of this throughout the organization could probably be detected in relationship to clients, other workers, and the administration.

The consultant really becomes a part of the system, even though he is not administratively within the organization. As he enters the organization he brings with him the possibility of either healing a dysfunctional split or perhaps producing one.

11. **Can you give me an example of how the consultant can act to correct a dysfunctional split?**

With a consultee (or group of consultees) he must use his clinical sense and note how the person presents himself. He must also be aware of whether he as consultant supports or rejects this presentation. The effective consultation position requires treating the consultee as competent to deal with the work problems objectively.

I recall a young school nurse who presented the case of an angry young boy who used to come to her office. While she was very irritated with this boy, she presented herself as a passive and accepting person who looked to me for a message from on high. In everything that I did in that consultation I tried to avoid both accepting this mantle and treating her as someone who did not have the resources to deal with this case. There are many subtle ways to create this effect, in the way that one sits and talks and especially in the way that one invites the consultee to participate.

12. **Can you give me an example of how this kind of activity on the part of the consultant might affect the whole organization?**

I recall a consultant who went to work in a newly funded and still disorganized agency. He very skillfully and thoughtfully spent a great amount of time with the people in the agency defining what his job would be. In the process of defining the limits of his role, it became absolutely necessary that those he talked to define *their* tasks, roles, and responsibilities. As this consultant described his experience, one could see that the organization had begun to coalesce around him, in the sense that his insistence on clarity for himself had helped others to define their roles and tasks.

At the opposite extreme, a consultant to a very rigid parochial school took a very casual attitude toward the contractual agreements and negotiations, indicating his trust that things would "work out." He believed he did not have to be too clear or definitive in what he said or did. The school was already overorganized. The consultees found in working with him that it was possible to let people act a little more freely than they had before. This organization absorbed the message he had brought and began to loosen up some of its rather rigid policies.

The consultant should retain some objectivity in his work with the consultee and not be caught in whatever dysfunctional stance the consultee presents. If the consultant is to be really helpful to the consultee he must retain his own neutral position, not accepting in his own view the helplessness and incompetence or, for that matter, the authoritarianism and supercompetence with which a consultee characterizes himself. He works toward an egalitarian, interdependent, trusting, and mutually respectful relationship.

13. **What you describe makes me think of the McLuhan statement that "the medium is the message."**

Well, it is a little like that. The stance that the consultant takes, his relationship to people in the organization, can be seen as the *medium* and at the same time may be one of the important *messages* he has to deliver to the organization and the people working in it.

---

exercises for chapter 7

1. In groups of three, one member should act as consultant, another

as consultee, and a third as observer.

The consultee is an elementary schoolteacher who presents the case of a hyperactive restless child who gets out of his seat at various times and disrupts the class. He takes so much of her time that she feels it interferes with her work with the other children. She feels a great sense of urgency about the case and wishes an "instant final solution" from the consultant in the form of a prescription for how to control the child's behavior or perhaps agreement that he should be transferred to another class. She says desperately, "I've got to do something with that child."

The consultant's task is to find a way to move the teacher, in her concern with the case, from the quest for an "instant final solution" toward an interest in the process characteristics of what goes on between her and this child. If she is to become interested in working further with this case, she will have to begin to see that there is something positive in the case for her. She will have to see that the problem is workable and that it can provide opportunity for her to grow and improve in her teaching skills.

Continue the dialogue between consultant and consultee for about five minutes. With the observer, discuss which elements of the consultation were successful and which were not.

Now change roles, with the consultant becoming the observer, the consultee the consultant, and the observer the consultee. Reenact the consultation, trying to use what was learned from the discussion. Then discuss what went on as before.

When you have completed the discussion, exchange roles once more. Again, the consultant becomes the observer, the observer the consultee, and the consultee becomes the consultant. Using what was learned from the second discussion, reenact the consultation again. Then discuss the whole process.

2. In each of the following cases, the distraught feelings of the consultee could easily be interpreted by a clinician as indicative of a personality disorder. The task of the consultant is to focus on the report of the consultee in such a way that it acknowledges whatever healthy role striving he can find. The consultant should readily acknowledge these as evidence of the consultee's competence.

In groups of three, each person should have an opportunity to be consultant and consultee at least once each.

A. A probation officer tells the consultant about a case in which he is angry. He berates his client for not adhering to the probation rules. Continue the dialogue.
B. A welfare worker is very angry at an unmarried mother of seven children who has just become pregnant again. Continue the dialogue.
C. A public health nurse has been criticized by her supervisor for spending excessive amounts of time with a young mother who has recently had back surgery. In the nurse's view, her patient's husband should be more sympathetic of her situation. In the supervisor's view, the nurse is overprotecting the patient, who should be doing more for herself and working toward greater independence. Continue the dialogue.

Discuss these three instances from the following standpoints:
A. Was the consultant able to find some healthy role-related striving to comment upon?
B. Were the comments unnatural and awkward, or did they seem genuine?
C. What might the consultant have said that would have achieved the same purpose but also felt natural and genuine?

Reenact the three consultations.

3. Divide in pairs. Engage in what was described in the text as the "definitional process:" differentiation of the role of the mental health professional from that of the consultee, and differentiation of the functions of the mental health program from those of the consultee agency. Try to engage in this as though it were a part of the consultation process. Consider the system differences, client differences, differences in perspective in the two agencies, differences in resources, and the different kinds of interventions that would be appropriate in each. Members of the pair should play consultant and consultee alternately in the following cases.

A. A probation officer discusses a young man recently out of jail on a narcotics charge. The probation officer is concerned that the young man may go back to drugs and wants to talk with the consultant about the things he can do to prevent this.
B. A schoolteacher describes a bright student who stutters.

She feels confident that the student is capable of superior work, but sometimes he seems to withdraw. She knows that sometimes the other children make fun of him.

C. A minister has been visiting a family with a young Mongoloid child. The family is very religious and wish spiritual help from him. The minister wants to be helpful but feels puzzled as to what he should do.

4. Break into groups of four, each forming a rhombus. The members of each group are an administrator or supervisor, a line worker, a client, and a consultant. The task is to simulate certain kinds of communication between the administrator, the worker, and the client. Do not involve the consultant yet.

In each case (given in detail below) the speaker should speak his piece to the second member. They should have a few minutes of conversational exchange, and then the receiver of the communication should deliver the message to the third member. There should be some conversational exchange, and then the third member should deliver the message back to the first member. Continue the discussion from person to person until either the supervisor or worker wishes consultation. Then the consultant should be called in and the problem discussed. Here are the examples:

A. An administrator in a welfare agency is very authoritarian. He never invites discussion by his workers. He simply lays down the law. The administrator conveys this message to the worker: You will have to cut out all of the recipients of aid who are over sixty years old. The worker then must tell his sixty-year-old client about this. The client then has access to the administrator. Take about two minutes for the discussion in each dialogue unit. Ask the consultant for help when you are ready.

B. A sanitarian has visited a local restaurant. The conditions are deplorable. In this health office the sanitarian must get the approval of his supervisor, the health officer, before he can bring pressure or close the restaurant. The sanitarian feels an urgency about doing something about this restaurant since he considers it a clear danger to the community. He goes to the health officer and tries to get him to make a decision. The health officer gives him a mixed and indecisive message. Play out that dialogue. Then the sanitarian goes to the restaurateur and discusses the problem with him. The restaurateur has access to the health officer and can then pick up the dialogue with him. After you have played out each of these dialogues for about two minutes, either the health officer or the sanitarian may request consultation.

C. An aggressive, very intelligent young man is on probation. He tells his probation officer that his brother is sick in a nearby state and urgently needs him. The conditions of his probation preclude his leaving the state. He tries to pressure the probation officer into getting special permission to let him go out of state. He even has a letter, allegedly from his brother, supporting his claim. The probation officer is aware that his own supervisor, from whom he would have to get permission, is a very passive and sometimes resistant person, and is unlikely to accede. Begin the dialogue with the client trying to pressure the probation officer. Continue as the probation officer tries to get approval from his supervisor. The client himself may also go directly to the supervisor at some point. Take about two minutes for each segment, and then ask for consultation.

5. This time break into groups of three. The discussion will be among a consultant, an administrator, and a staff worker. All of them meet together.

A. A police precinct, widely known as the most tightly organized, rigid organization of its kind, has recently had a lot of trouble. The lieutenant in charge of the precinct has, through a regular police channel, requested mental health consultation. The consultant meets with the lieutenant and one of the sergeants. Their dialogue reflects the tight character of the organization. The negotiations for the contract for the consultation are very precise and authoritarian from the standpoint of the police department. Continue the dialogue as the consultant tries to get involved in the consultation project.

B. A consultant gets a written request from the regional administrator of an OEO program to go to a newly formed agency providing work training in a ghetto area. The letter simply says that arrangements have been made for the consultation and that he can arrive at his convenience at the office. The address is listed. The administrator also indicates that there is some urgency about the consultation but gives no name of a contact person. The consultant tries to follow up on this with a telephone call to the administrator, but the administrator is in Washington for several months. He talks to a deputy who only knows that the agency "really needs consultation" and that they would be very appreciative of the consultant's help. Everything is very hazy and unstructured. The consultant, after discussing this with his program administrator, decides that, despite the odd character of the request, it is worthwhile trying to get started since this is an important agency. The consultant goes to the agency, which he finds very disorganized. After a lengthy search, he finds someone identified as the administrator of the agency. When he asks this man if this is so, the man says, "I guess so, but I'm not really sure." Also present is a man identified as a staff member. Pick up the dialogue among all three of these as the consultant tries to establish some limits for the consultation program.

Afterwards, discuss the experience from these standpoints:

1) What was the "parallel process" and how was it manifested?
2) What kinds of messages were implicitly and explicitly conveyed to the system by the consultant's behavior, statements, and questions?

CHAPTER 8

Some Specific Elements of Mental Health Consultation

1. I have a reasonably clear picture of the broad outlines of mental health consultation, I think, and how it relates to and affects the social systems. I also have a good idea of how to keep the process related to the structures set up for it. You have given me a sense of the flow of the process through beginning, middle, and end, and I think I now understand the crucial timing issues. You have also described the working concept and the nonspecific elements of consultation. I feel ready now for some of the specific methods of consultation you promised.

   That is a clear summary of where you are and a good lead-in to some of the specific elements of mental health consultation. These elements are specific in the sense that they are designed to meet special needs of the consultee. As such, they depend on how the consultant understands and diagnoses the consultee's needs. I think of the needs in three general categories.

   A. *Information and knowledge* that you possess as a mental health professional and that will help him in carrying out his job.

    B. *Skills:* knowing what to do and how. This knowledge, which the consultant has as a mental health professional, may be shared to help the consultee with some aspect of his job.

    C. *Help with an attitudinal block,* when there is something in a case which keeps the consultee from effectively using himself or the resources available to him to do his job.

2. **Let's begin with the first category. What kind of information and knowledge does the mental health professional have which can help the consultee do his job better?**

    You recall that we made quite a point of the difference in the backgrounds of the consultant and consultee. Each has some special competence to bring to bear on the problem of the consultation. You will recall that in the first lesson you were asked to list the things in which you were an expert. Your expertise and competence are derived from the knowledge and skill you've acquired in your own training. Most commonly, this means clinical knowledge, although, as we will see it, is not necessarily limited to clinical considerations. Here are some examples of situations in which mental health consultants may have some information that would be useful to a consultee:

    A. A welfare worker is concerned about the suicidal risk of an elderly man who has begun to speak vaguely of dying. He is chronically ill with the complications of diabetes and his wife died two months ago.

    B. A minister is concerned about a single lady, aged fifty-two, who has been one of his parishioners over twenty years. Recently, she told him that some of the men in the congregation were making obscene gestures to her.

    C. A welfare worker has had a new case transferred to her. He is a post-hospital schizophrenic patient who has been living in a board and care home for over a year. The first time she interviewed him, he casually mentioned that he was actively involved in arms reduction talks with the Soviet Union and that he was in close communication daily with the Pentagon. This information frightened her, as she had never seen anyone quite like him before. She wonders if he should go back to the hospital.

    D. A welfare worker has had a new patient added to her case

load. He has been recently released from a state hospital. Although in his discussion with her he seemed pleasant and realistic, he complained to her of great feelings of restlessness and during their meeting he jumped up from his chair several times and walked about, seemingly without reason. She also noted that several times he seemed to be drooling. She wants to discuss what this may mean.

E. A minister tells the consultant of his concern for a man whose wife of eight years was killed in an automobile accident three weeks ago. The minister says that the man has been doing a great deal of crying and says that, "Life is not worth living." He has not been working. The minister wants to know if this is a normal reaction or if it is pathological.

F. A fourth-grade teacher had a child enter her class when the family moved to the community three months ago. The child was an excellent student and seemed to make a good adjustment. It is now nearly the end of the term and suddenly his work has fallen off and he has spoken to the teacher about the fact that he does not want to be promoted to Miss Miller's class with the other children. She wants to know if this is abnormal or not.

G. The same schoolteacher wants to know if there is any place in the community without a long waiting list to which she could refer such a child, if it were indicated, for psychiatric help.

3. These are all items on which I could provide some useful information, on the basis of what I learned in my basic clinical work. Can you discuss important factors in the *manner* in which a consultant should give such information?

There are several points to consider. First, as you can see, in nearly all of the examples listed above there is some ambiguity. More information is needed. A certain amount of exploration is almost always needed to get the necessary facts. Then you can determine what information is useful and whether the information you have is appropriate to the case. The more the consultant can learn about the situation, the more likely it is that he will be able to answer the consultee's needs competently.

A second point concerns the amount of information to be given. There is a great temptation for a consultant to give a lengthy discourse. Some of the information may be pertinent and some not. Too much information may be difficult for the consultee to handle or may be confusing. The consultant should try to be as specific as possible in what he offers.

Sometimes the mental health professional may have conflicting bodies of information and may want to allow the consultee to select what he wishes. The consultant may see this as in keeping with the model of consultation which we have presented. However, it should be emphasized that allowing the consultee the freedom of choice in what he takes away from the consultation does not diminish the consultant's responsibility for the pertinence of what he offers.

The final point has to do with timing and where to stop. Because there is such a welter of information in the mental health field (some of it fascinating, some of it conflicting) and because we are sometimes appropriately modest about the level of our scientific accuracy, a consultant sometimes will keep giving information to a consultee beyond the point of usefulness, precluding any sense of closure for the consultee. The consultant may leave the session feeling that he has "given his all," but the consultee may leave confused and dissatisfied because he does not know what to do with what he has heard.

4. I feel quite secure about information related to clinical activities, but what if the consultant is working with an administrator on information related to administrative issues?

Mental health professionals are often called upon to provide consultation on administrative matters. Some may take the position that they can help the administrator with his personal dilemma around an administrative issue without having any special knowledge of administration. This may be true, but I would encourage any consultant who enters into such a consultation to be very clear in his own mind about the limits of his knowledge. As for myself, in order to be comfortable in such a situation, I would have to declare openly to the consultee which areas I knew something about and which I did not.

We have seen some real disasters in situations where the consultant got into a relationship with a consultee who expected him to be an administrative expert and the consultant accepted the mantle without its being warranted. The problems of administration are as complex and demanding as the problems of clinical practice, and if we really respect these we should treat them accordingly.

5. **As you talk about it, I realize that there are a number of areas outside of clinical training of which a mental health professional might have some special knowledge.**

That is right. He may have some special knowledge and skill in the area of social welfare. This, of course, is particularly true of psychiatric social workers. He may be an expert in research and evaluation. Often psychologists have these skills. Similarly, psychologists sometimes have a special competence in education. Social workers may know about community organization. Physicians, of course, have their medical training, as do nurses. A clinician coming from any of the disciplines may have developed a special competence in group work. If a consultation program has more than one consultant available, it is well to try to match the consultant with the consultee's need during the negotiation period.

6. **I think I am ready now to go on to the next category of need: when the consultee's desire is for** *skill.*

This, of course, is closely related to the matter of giving the appropriate information. In each case a mental health professional is experienced in the specific problem and knows something about how to handle it.

Let's consider the example 2A above, in which the elderly man is clearly a suicidal risk. The important activity might be to find ways of mobilizing a human support system: i.e., facilitating friendships and contacting family members if they are available.

In example 2B, the probably involutional woman of concern to the minister, referral to a mental health program *might* be an important action. Ways of doing this could be discussed.

In example 2C, concerning the post-hospital schizophrenic patient, it could be clarified that a decision about the hospitalization should not be made on the basis of his delusions but on the capability of the individual to function in his specific social setting. This might require the worker to gather additional supportive information. The consultant would want to inquire about the patient's strengths as well as psychopathology.

The post-hospital patient in example 2D would appear to be having some side effects from drugs. After this is determined, appropriate action would be recommended and taken.

7. **What are the special things to look for in offering a method of doing something?**

The first thing to keep in mind is that the goal of consultation is not to make the consultee into a psychotherapist or caseworker. The goal is not to reeducate him so that he will become another mental health professional; rather it is to provide him with certain knowledge and skills which he can *translate* into his own social system and tasks. Thus, the consultant must make sure that what he offers or suggests in terms of action is translated into the definitional characteristics of the consultee's job. If a particular suggestion cannot be translated, and frequently this is the case, it should be rejected and a new mode of action considered which will fit into the consultee's perspective.

It is tempting for a consultant to become a teacher of psychotherapy, particularly if the consultee appears to be an eager pupil. With a commitment to psychotherapy a mental health worker may tend to overlook the importance of the consultee's job. However, even if the consultee became a skilled psychotherapist, then someone new would have to be hired to do his job in the consultee organization. Moreover, the consultee would likely be dissatisfied with his job instead of feeling an increased sense of satisfaction and valuing it.

8. **Wait a minute! If the consultant is talking to the consultee about how to handle a case, he may be getting into the *supervisory* process, and so breaking a rule stated earlier.**

I am pleased that you brought that up. It still holds true that the consultee and his supervisor, and not the consultant, are the ones who are accountable for what goes on in the agency. As you detected, talking about what the consultee should do is a potential hazard for the consultant. In highly sophisticated agencies there may be considerably less need for this focus in consultation, as supervisors may take care of a good deal of it. Nevertheless, the mental health consultant does have special knowledge and skill in dealing with the mental health aspects of the consultee's case load. A transgression into supervision will not occur so long as the consultant clearly has in mind what the limits of his role are. In discussing any action, he must raise questions about what is acceptable in the agency, whether the supervisor has been involved in the discussions, and the details of the agency structure: all things that we have been discussing. The consultant may have some important information to offer on what to do, but it must be translated by the consultee into his own professional frame of reference. The consultee must be clearly aware that accountability and responsibility have not been taken from him as a result of the consultant's suggestions, and that it is still up to him and his supervisor to decide what is acceptable and not acceptable within the agency.

9. **I am ready now for a specific approach when the problem is the consultee's attitudinal block. But, first, isn't that just a euphemism for psychopathology?**

It would be if our concern were the personal functioning of the consultee. But that is not our focus. We are interested in what the consultee needs in order to do his job, and so we are also interested in anything that might interfere with his doing it as well as he might. Our contract is not to help him to be a better or more fulfilled person, but to be more effective in his job. Of course, he is likely to feel more fulfilled if he does a better job.

10. **I see your point. I am surprised how difficult it is for me as a clinician to stay within the job focus. I keep slipping into my clinical stance and looking for intrapsychic conflicts. Let's go on.**

The attitudinal block can be seen as something which keeps the consultee from using his full potential. Something limits him. An example of this is the "theme interference," which Gerald Caplan has described so competently. Essential to the concept of theme interference is stereotyping. When a consultee, or anyone else for that matter, stereotypes someone else, it is likely to be dehumanizing. What the consultee sees and hears is not another live, breathing human being, but a stereotype. His attitude toward the stereotype is predetermined and how he behaves is likely also to be stereotyped. He is not able to see his client as he is and he is not able to work with him with his full capacity.

11. **That is really translating psychopathology into job functioning terms. I like that, but I am not so sure that it is necessary.**

    One thing we know from research in psychology is that something has to give if you think one way and behave another (Festinger and Frank). There is a natural, healthy tendency in humans to synthesize and integrate incongruencies in thought and speech or action. In this case, it is hard to "think pathology" and "talk health" to the consultee. The consultant needs concepts which are consistent for his thought and action.

12. **Yes. Now please continue your discussion of stereotyping.**

    A stereotype is a cliché. Once a person is identified this way, it is as though nothing more need be said; it is complete. An example is the statement that "all white (black) (yellow) people look alike." We are all aware of how such stereotypes inhibit human interactions.

13. **Then you are talking about stereotypes that people have as members of a particular reference group?**

    There are two kinds of stereotypes and the group type is one. Group-based stereotypes are those which have special meaning in a particular consultee agency, profession, or system. They are shared by most or all of the people in the agency, and they are usually rationalized.

    For example, in medicine, the term "crock" is applied to some chronic patients, and once this happens there is a feeling of hopelessness about being able to help. Physicians tend to avoid them and in clinics they are often transferred from service to service. It is as though there is nothing more to be said or done once a person has been so stereotyped.

    Sometimes a series of euphemisms is applied to try to break a stereotype, but soon the euphemism becomes only another symbol for it. In psychiatry, changing the name of "back wards" to "chronic wards" to "continuous treatment wards" had little effect on the essential stereotype.

    The other kind of stereotype is a personal one and relates to something unique to the consultee. These stereotypes tend to be largely unconscious and must be inferred by the consultant. As an example, I remember a school nurse who had great concern about "show-offs." For several weeks running, she talked about different children who were "show-offs." Wherever she looked, she seemed to find them.

Of course the degree of stereotyping is strongly affected by social and individual factors and may be in varying degrees both conscious and unconscious.

14. **Well, I understand what a stereotype is, but I am not clear about how that relates to theme interference.**

In Caplan's concept, theme interference is composed of a stereotype and a prediction of outcome, usually bad. For example, in the case of the "crocks" they are "beyond help" and doomed to be the pariahs of the medical care system. In the case of the nurse who was concerned about "show-offs," the outcome she "knew" would occur was that "show-offs" would not be liked by others and they would be ostracized and left alone. The stereotype may become a self-fulfilling prophecy as the feelings engendered in the consultee drive him away from the client.

15. **In a way, couldn't you say that learning to be a mental health professional, or any other kind of professional, is a matter of learning stereotypes, of learning how to categorize things and learning certain kinds of expected outcomes? I don't see that that is necessarily bad.**

There is a similarity. The difference is whether or not the stereotyping limits or expands the helping activities and attitudes of the worker. If it is simply a shorthand which allows him to be more efficient under certain circumstances, that is all to the good, but if he mistakes the symbols and the shorthand for the human being he is working with and, in addition, anticipates that nothing can be done, the consultee is severely limited in doing his job.

16. **I can see that. Could you say something more about how to identify a stereotype and theme interference?**

Well, we have talked about some of the characteristics, such as having a cliché (like "show-off") attached to the stereotype. The person is described as though nothing more need be said about him once he has been placed in the category. When a consultant begins to inquire for details of a stereotyped case he may find that the consultee has great difficulty in substantiating the stereotype. The details may be vague or in some way incongruent. There is also the narrowness of the description: it is two-dimensional. The client is seen only in terms of the stereotype and its negative qualities. No strengths are described to round it out. Finally, upon inquiry, you can usually learn something of the disastrous outcome anticipated for the client by the consultee.

17. **I think I can recognize the theme interference now. How can I handle it?**

The consultant can handle this problem on several lines, as follows:

A. *The nonverbal focus on the case.* The consultant does not panic and he does not share the despair or frustration experienced by the consultee. He indicates by his manner simply that he would calmly like to examine the evidence. This is reassuring to the consultee and motivates him to look anew at the case.

B. *The nonverbal focus on the consultant-consultee relationship.* Here the consultant uses his clinical skills to see if there is a parallel between the way the consultee presents himself to the consultant and the way the consultee describes the client. The consultant will wish to maintain the relationship of two colleagues and to indicate his confidence in the competence of the consultee to handle the situation. This is as we described it before when we discussed the parallel process.

C. *Verbal examination of the evidence.* The consultant focuses verbally on the case, raising questions to reveal whether or not the anticipated tragic outcome in the theme interference follows from a more detailed description of the case. The consultant does not challenge the stereotyped category in which the consultee places the client, but tries through his questions and observations to determine if there are not alternative outcomes that could occur.

18. **I don't really understand the purpose of this. Aren't you interested in changing the stereotype?**

Yes. However, if the consultee leaves consultation with the idea that only this *particular* client does not fall into the stereotyped category, it does not diminish the likelihood that he will stereotype another client in the same way. What has been accomplished under these circumstances is that there has been an unlinking; that is, the stereotype is seen as the invalid in this particular case *only*. The "bad outcome" is still considered to follow inevitably from the stereotype by the consultee. This may be useful for the particular case but does not liberate the consultee from future stereotyping in similar cases. The consultant hopes that as he works with a consultee the whole theme will diminish. This way, the consultant has not only assisted the consultee in his capacity to deal with this case, but also in his capacity to deal with other similar cases.

19. **I can see that point as being useful in the long run. Incidentally, it certainly is apparent to me that the methods for reducing a specific theme interference are consistent with what you described earlier in the process and generic methods.**

Yes, they are the same methods. The difference is that here they are focused on case material with a specific conceptualization and outcome in mind: the reduction of the theme interference.

Both the generic and the more specific approaches to consultation are aspects of the art of inquiry. The consultant orients himself, and thereby the consultee, toward understanding as fully as possible both the client as a whole person and the whole system. The consultant assumes that behind the selective perceptions of the consultee about the client (his stereotype) there is more. He assumes that the consultee is stuck because he is seeing only a part of the client and utilizing only a part of his own resources and potential. He has stereotyped not only the client and his needs, but also his own capability to relate and be helpful. The consultant by his inquiry seeks to liberate the consultee from the limitations of selective perception. The solutions will, he hopes, follow naturally.

As an example, the consultee often will present the problem client to the consultant with a statement such as, "What do you do about troublemakers?" The consultant, at that point, will not wish to enter into a general discussion about what might be done about troublemakers. Instead, he will want to learn all that he can about the whole person who has been labeled in this way. As he inquires, the troublemaker can be seen more as a human being capable of responding to human contact. This opens new opportunities for the consultee to do his work effectively.

20. **Is there anything else the consultant can do or say that might help to reduce theme interference?**

Sometimes one can make a general statement in opposition to the linkage between the stereotype and the outcome, but this is not usually very effective. Another means is what Caplan calls the "parable technique." The consultant tells a story from his own experience or another source in which the predicted outcome did not follow from the stereotype.

21. **If you want to show that the outcome anticipated by the consultee doesn't necessarily follow from the stereotype, another way occurs to me as a possibility. Why not just see the client yourself as a consultant, and then discuss your findings with the consultee, emphasizing those which do not confirm the "bad outcome" prediction?**

Very good. That is a useful method and one which sometimes fits the situation better than others. It should certainly be one of the methods available to the consultant.

22. **Another useful method might be to invite a group of consultees to make observations about a potential outcome. They might become allies to the consultant in his work.**

Yes, they might. Group members, particularly if they know something about the case, can supply very important information that may reduce the theme interference. The group may serve as important allies in this process. In addition, since the theme may have strong system implications, the involvement of the group may have important effects throughout the organization.

Caplan has expressed the concern that in a group one member may see an unconscious personal conflict within the presenting consultee and confront him with it. This may have the undesirable effect that we have stressed of reducing the consultee's confidence and competence to do the job. However, most group members identify with the consultant's respectful attitude toward the consultee and his dilemma and so avoid destructive comments. Moreover, the consultant may insure this by his keeping the focus clearly on the client being discussed and by structuring the discussion so that it is directed initially toward *understanding the case* rather than toward finding solutions. If he can focus the group's attention in this way, he may avoid blaming or confrontation. He may even wish to emphasize that the focus is not on determining what is good or bad in the case but on understanding in a nonjudgmental way.

The "safety valve" for the consultant is in always being able to return to the focus: the task on which the group has agreed to work. In most situations the focus is the case, but it can also be a program or a supervisee. Some groups may require that the consultant monitor activities a little more closely than others in order to keep the case from becoming a discussion of the consultee's psychopathology.

23. **I wonder if we could go through an example of theme interference reduction step by step. I think I understand it, but this would help.**

Some examples are shown on the charts which follow. They should clarify the whole procedure.

THEME INTERFERENCE AND REDUCTION
Individual Theme

Consultee: Elementary school nurse, newly employed. She is a new member of an ongoing group of nurse consultees.

Client: What do you do about "show offs?" Case: An eight-year-old girl.

Stereotyped initial category: "Show off"

Prediction of outcome: Will be disliked and ostracized, left alone.

Consultant's activity:

1. *Nonverbal focus on cases:* Consultant not in despair or panic about case. Discusses case calmly and objectively.

2. *Nonverbal focus on relationship:* Consultee is attractive, talkative, very brightly dressed. Immediately takes center of group and dramatically presents case while closely noting other group members' reactions to her. Consultant wonders at parallel between her behavior in group and description of client. He is careful to be objective and professional, treating her as a competent equal. He also attempts to facilitate common interest of presenter with other consultees.

(left margin, vertical text) "Theme interference" stereotype and outcome linked inevitably

3. *Verbal examination of evidence:* Inquiry shows that client is not ostracized and is quite popular with her peers.
4. *Verbal parable technique:* "She reminds me of a little girl I once knew in a nursery school. She was a 'show off' but she was also able to have some very close friendships."
5. *Verbal direct state of generalization:* Because someone is a "show off" he will not necessarily be ostracized.
6. *Verbal joint observation and discussion:* Consultant arranges to observe child in classroom and notes some evidence of warm relationships with others. He shares his observation with consultee.
7. *Group effects:* Group members are united as colleagues in common concern. Presenter is not alone.

GROUP INTERFERENCE AND REDUCTION

Group Theme

"Theme interference" stereotype and outcome linked inevitably

Consultees: Group of clinic physicians frustrated at not being able to help.

Client: Complain about "crock" – Consultant asks to discuss example.

Stereotyped initial category: "Crock" – a chronic hypochondriacal patient.

Prediction of outcome: They are leaches on others and can't be helped.

Consultant's activity:

1. *Nonverbal focus on cases:* Consultant brings hope. Objectively, without frustration, examines problem with colleagues.
2. *Nonverbal focus on relationship:* By his behavior, consultant treats consultees as colleagues capable of doing what is useful. Does not accept helplessness.
3. *Verbal examination of evidence:* Inquiry with group shows that patient is more than a stereotype, a "crock;" that he has many specific problems and assets and that there are avenues of treatment which might be useful.
4. *Verbal parable technique:* "I once knew a patient like this, with different outcome."
5. *Verbal direct statement of generalization:* "Chronic patients are not necessarily beyond help."
6. *Verbal joint observation and discussion:* Sees patient with doctor and discusses potential outcomes that are not necessarily bad.
7. *Group effect:* Share concern and begin to recall some of cases where good results were achieved.

24. I find theme interference particularly interesting and much like clinical work. I can use the skills that I have already developed—listening to the unconscious, noting nonverbal cues, and speaking to the unconscious in metaphors.

Yes, this method does appeal greatly to clinicians for those reasons, and it is a valuable part of consultation. But one should not be dazzled by it or trapped into viewing it as the *only* part of consultation. It is one effective method, but the others we have discussed are equally important. Some of the more obvious things which may not require as much subtlety, such as giving information or maintaining links with the system, may be the most effective and important tools in consultation. It is important not to lose sight of the forest while looking at the trees: this is a temptation with theme interference reduction.

---

exercises for chapter 8

Practice sessions will deal with some of the examples given in the text above. The following exercises may be done in pairs with one member as consultant and the other as consultee, or in a group situation with one member as consultant, another as the presenter, and the others as members of a consultee group.

1. In each of the following cases, begin the dialogue with the consultee's description of the problem. Then take a couple of minutes for the consultant to explore some more details. The consultant should then spend about five minutes in discussion with the consultee, *giving him information* which will help him to understand the case. Then discuss for a few minutes what went on in each case.

The times given for completing the exercises are, of course, arbitrary. In a real consultation session such time limitations would not be imposed. Limiting the times would encourage the consultant to be concise and focused in his activities. In a real situation he would have an opportunity to be much more thorough. The exercise is solely for the purpose of illustrating the issues involved.

A. A welfare worker is concerned over the suicidal risk of an elderly man who has begun to speak vaguely of dying. He is chronically ill with the residuals of diabetes, and his wife died two months ago.

B. A minister is concerned about a single lady, aged fifty-two, who has been one of his parishioners over twenty years. Recently she told him that some of the men in the congregation were making obscene gestures to her.

C. A welfare worker has had a new case transferred to her. He is a post-hospital schizophrenic patient who has been living in a board and care home for over a year. The first time she interviewed him, he casually mentioned that he was actively involved in arms reduction talks with the Soviet Union and that he was in close communication daily with the Pentagon. This information frightened her, as she had never seen anyone quite like him before. She wonders if he should go back to the hospital.

D. A welfare worker has had a new client added to her case load who is recently released from a state hospital. Although in his discussion with her he seemed pleasant and realistic, he complained to her of great feelings of restlessness and during their meeting he seemingly without reason jumped up from his chair and walked about several times. She also noted that several times he seemed to be drooling. She wants to discuss the meaning of this.

E. A minister tells the consultant of his concern for a man whose wife of eight years was killed in an automobile accident three weeks ago. The minister says that the man has been doing a great deal of crying and says that "Life is not worth living." He has not been working. The minister wants to know if this is a normal reaction or if it is pathological.

F. A fourth-grade schoolteacher had a child enter her class when the family moved to the community three months ago. The child was an excellent student and seemed to make a good adjustment. It is nearly the end of the term and suddenly his work has fallen off. He has spoken to the teacher about the fact that he does not want to be promoted to Miss Miller's class with the other children. She wants to know if this is abnormal or not.

2. Now take about five minutes during which the consultant will discuss with the consultee *what action* might appropriately be taken to deal with the situation. Then take a few minutes to discuss what went on in each case.

3. Again use the case material above. The consultant has now provided the consultee with the information to understand the case. After exploration of courses of action, a preliminary plan has been decided upon, but a new element enters into the consultation process. The consultant becomes aware of an attitudinal block in the consultee which inhibits him from utilizing his understanding and which blocks him from appropriately following a course of action. The consultant begins to note a theme interference and now his task is to spend about five minutes working toward the reduction of that interference.

    A. The consultee says, "The poor man (referring to example 1A above). I keep thinking about him all the time, when I am with other clients and then when I go home at night. It just seems so sad and so hopeless. I've got to do something for him right now."

In the simulation the consultee should pick up this dialogue, and the consultant should respond.

    B, C, D, E, F. In each case the consultee should take a minute or so to identify with the appropriate description in exercise 1. He should then try to establish a "set" in which he has overidentified with his client. When he has established this in his mind, he should pick up the consultation with the consultant. Again the consultant's task is to work toward the reduction of the theme interference.

On the completion of each of the cases, discuss the consultation process from the standpoint of the following:

    A. Which of the methods described in the text above were used?

    B. Was there any evidence of change in the consultee's attitude?

    C. Did the consultant challenge the stereotype or did he

confine his activities as described in the text to working on the prediction of outcome?

4. One member of the group should be the consultant and several others should be members of the consultee group. The session is an early meeting of the consultant with a group of third-grade teachers. He is endeavoring to understand some of the main problems faced by the teachers. One of the teachers says that she has a "hyperactive child" in her class. The other teachers all respond knowingly. Just the mention of the hyperactive child seems to trigger something in them. There are several groans and a general sense of futility is expressed. The consultant senses a group stereotype here. His task is to work toward the reduction of this stereotype. Begin the dialogue.

5. This is again a group situation, with one member as a consultant and the others as a group of physical education teachers in an early session. One teacher mentions the problem with "non-strip" cases. The consultant is puzzled and does not understand what is meant. All of the teachers indicate recognition of the syndrome and its hopelessness. As the consultant inquires, it turns out that a "non-strip" is a student who does not change into gym clothes. He always has an excuse so that he doesn't have to. The teachers are frustrated and angry about them. Begin the dialogue at this point.

6. A consultant is telephoned by the principal of a school where he has been consulting with several groups of teachers. The consultant has dropped into the principal's office when he could and has done a good job of maintaining his link with the administration. Now the principal calls him and says he has a serious problem about which he would like to talk to the consultant. They arrange an appointment in the principal's office for later that day. The consultant senses the urgency of this meeting.

The principal begins by saying, "It's these damned militants again." Four black teachers in his school have sent him a petition saying that they will no longer use the textbook required by law in his school. They say that it expresses "racist" attitudes and that they can no longer use it. They say that they plan to devote the time that would be used on the study of this textbook to "black studies." This has not been defined. The classes of these teachers are roughly half black and half white.

Begin the dialogue and continue it for about five minutes.

7. A consultant has been working with the officers of a probation department. He has had a cordial but distant relationship with the administrator. On one of his regular visits, as he often does, he stops by the administrator's office for a brief contact. The administrator says, "Boy, am I glad to see you! I've got a problem I've got to talk to somebody about. Do you have some time?" The consultant has a group meeting scheduled in five minutes. He is very much aware of the time as the administrator continues to go on, saying that one of his supervisors, who has up to now been very competent and able, has told his workers that they should no longer obey a probation rule which forbids probationees from leaving the country without permission. He has told his workers that is is an "unfair" rule. He has then sent a note to the administrator telling him what has been done, but has not come to see him personally.

Begin the dialogue at this point. Afterward discuss what went on.

CHAPTER 9

Mental Health Education

1. You have been saying often that mental health consultation is *not* education. I do not really understand. In a mental health consultation, don't you expect the consultee to learn something? Why else would he return?

Your question is indeed valid. A consultee gets help with his dilemma and in the course of the consultation may learn new interpretations or new facts about his problem, his agency, or the community. I call such learning a secondary gain of the *consultation* process. I admit I have a bias about this in calling it a secondary gain, but as a teacher of mental health consultation I have frequently seen a consultant concentrate so much on the teaching of case dynamics and the elaboration of psychological significances that he paid little attention to the central matter of his consultee's dilemma over his situation. Knowing more facts *may* free a person to act, but not necessarily so. Being freer to act may not necessarily be tied to acquiring more facts.

2. What, specifically, goes into the helping aspect as opposed to the educational aspect?

What goes into the process of helping the consultee is all the elements that we have presented in previous chapters; careful entry into the consultee system; well understood mutual agreements regarding purpose and structure; renegotiation of purpose, structure and methods with consultees; clarification of the consultant's role; maintenance of focus; and initiation and sustenance of the interactive process in time. The consultant provides essential help with the consultee's dilemma in giving understanding and facilitating response to blockings and/or apprehensions that could cloud the consultee's vision and warp his decisions for activity.

3. **I think I see what you mean. Mental health consultation is in some ways like the therapeutic situation, but it is also very different in that it deals with work groups, social systems, and even the community. It also differs in its narrower objectives and specific task orientation.**

Yes. Psychotherapy generally deals with the whole self and tries to help with diverse aspects of a person's life. Mental health consultation deals with more than one person and deals only with a particular work problem which may be set within a large system of interlocking work relationships. In each situation, the psychotherapist or consultant uses all his understanding of individual psychodynamics and group interrelationships, but he *acts* on his knowledge *differently,* in accord with the different objectives of the two processes.

4. **I think I now understand more fully the differences between psychotherapy and mental health consultation. What are your ideas on mental health *education?***

A number of mental health centers have a staff member designated as Mental Health Educator. In other centers many staff members carry responsibilities in mental health education.

We need to start from the same base of role definition, functions, and expectations of both the learner and teacher. Almost everyone working in the mental health field has experienced many years of prescribed schooling. We have mixed feelings about teachers, and many of us may have reservations about being in either the learning or teaching role again.

5. **Granting that, can you tell me more about the process of mental health education?**

In a mental health educational project the teacher organizes what he knows about a given topic and presents it for the intellectual and perhaps emotional grasp of a lay group. Such students expect the teacher not only to know the subject and how to teach it, but also to be able to evaluate how well it has been learned. For example, in our study of consultation, one pivotal idea is to treat a consultee with respect for his competence and integrity as a worker. As a teacher, I think I could tell if a trainee had intellectually grasped that concept. Only with some effort in putting it into practice can it be *integrated* fully into the student's activity with consultees; however, I think it is unlikely that a person could achieve the second goal, integration into action, if he had not already achieved the first goal, the intellectual grasp of the idea. Hence the importance of mental health education.

6. **But isn't the *intellectual* grasp of material simply like reading a book? I think that method could be pretty sterile and not provide much real understanding of mental health.**

Yes, it *can* be like that, and is that way for some people on whom the teacher makes no impact. If the teacher can relate to the lay group and *involve* its members in the process of learning some dynamic concepts, the method can be fruitful and rewarding.

7. **You make it sound interesting, but hard! How do you do that? How do you go about it?**

The first action is essentially the entry phase described earlier. In this negotiating process with the administrator, it is important to clarify what sort of program is wanted. Is the aim to help people on specific job problems and questions, or to increase the knowledge base of the workers?

8. **But suppose they ask for mental health education with the idea that the staff will be "transformed" and thus will not need specific case consultation? If consultation is what they need, should you not press for that, or at least suggest it, as a better project for them?**

I think that decision must be made individually by each

mental health professional. I would rather respond by giving what a group wants, if I can. Of course, often what they want is not clear even to them; part of the contract negotiation is to help to focus and define the need clearly.

Many joint endeavors between caretaking agencies and mental health centers begin with mental health education projects and move naturally, in time, to mental health consultation projects. When a welfare system has developed enough trust in a mental health center staff member to seek mental health consultation on work problems, it has already moved a good distance toward constructive use of consultative help.

9. **Do you mean that the purpose of mental health education is, or could be, to get people to accept mental health consultation?**

No, I think that mental health education is a valid and profitable activity in itself, even if it never leads to mental health consultation. Through the negotiation process the agency clarifies its needs and the consultant outlines what he can offer that may possibly meet those needs.

10. **Even if administrators plan mental health education for their staffs, I should think it would be difficult to arouse real interest in a theoretical course. Welfare workers and probation officers generally have more to do in a week than they have time for. Why should they take on such a class?**

It is not easy, as you say. I can talk of several ways I've tried to work for interest and involvement in learning, and you may think of others.

A. During the negotiation period, I have suggested that *volunteers* sign up for a mental health education project.

B. If the administrator does not accept this suggestion, I say directly that the field of mental health is so large that it would be important in my planning for me to discuss with a small committee of staff members what topics and questions would be most pertinent to their work. This is generally easy to arrange. With such a committee, the mental health educator starts to work for their involvement in a joint plan.

C. Another thing I've done is ask the administrator if some supervisor would be willing to collect from each member a short paragraph delineating a topic or a work situation which he would like to understand more clearly. I have asked for these one week ahead of starting date. Generally I do not get a paper from each member, but I have always gotten something to start with.

D. A variation on C is to ask that each member mail his note to me directly. However, I generally do not get as good results with this.

E. One can also use the first session of the project to collect such topics and problems. It is helpful to talk of the mental health field in a general way. Try not to overrate or underrate it. I have found it useful to indicate that some of our knowledge is well accepted experientially, and well documented, some is theoretical, and some is merely fashionable — and that we do not have as yet, an accepted classical science of human behavior.

F. I think it is helpful to plan for a definite number of sessions within a specific calendar period. It is more propitious for learning to develop a second project than to continue a first one indefinitely.

It is important to distinguish between *learning about* behavior, attitudes, and emotions, and developing skill and proficiency in *dealing with* problem behavior. The educational project focuses upon "learning about," even though the students and I know that questions will come out of day-to-day work and that we will certainly be thinking about the practical implications of the material.

11. Suppose you get no suggestions for topics?

That could happen, but generally one gets some response, even if only from those who feel uncomfortable with a few seconds of silence. I try to make the most of anything offered, even building a topic out of a tangential remark. If no suggestions come, I might say that while they were thinking I could throw out some that might be pertinent. If it were a teacher group: "the young child just starting to school," "the middle years of childhood," "the teenager," "the child who does *not* use all his capacities," or "the truant child." If it were a probation group: "the first offender," "the young offender away from home," etc.

12. **It seems to me you are doing all the work! You ask them to suggest topics but if they don't you do.**

I guess it does look like that. If there is great resistance to moving into a required educational project, I think that this much work and contribution on the part of the teacher may demonstrate his willingness to help them even though they have no choice about being there.

13. **Wouldn't it be good to talk to them about that very situation?**

Yes, that might be helpful, but in a first experience with a group, it might also lead to a stalemate about an educational project. I would prefer to ask if the specific concrete items of time and place were inconvenient for many of them, and I would try to accommodate them in any way I could.

14. **I feel overwhelmed by the possibility of such resistance. Aren't there some people who want to learn?**

Yes, and with ordinary luck, you'll have a few of them in your group. If in the first session you work on the selection of topics, there is another point on which you can encourage their participation. The students can help you to rank order them, or at least star a few that should not be missed. In such a group discussion of priorities I myself have sometimes indicated *one* that I thought should not be missed, demonstrating *joint* planning and work.

If, however, short papers on topics and questions have been sent *ahead,* it is important to work on them *prior* to the session. They often lend themselves to groupings and suggest interrelated topics. With the use of a blackboard to show the spread of topics and the possible groupings, the discussion of priorities can go on as above.

15. **I can see that these methods might encourage more of a learning stance. Would you start to lecture right then?**

Before we focus on developing the content, let's stop over that word, "lecture." The word generally calls up a picture like its dictionary definition: "a formal discourse intended for instruction." I imagine you would agree that this reflects the antithesis of involved learning. The "lecture-discussion" or the "lecture-seminar" is the most frequent medium for mental health education. A few important considerations follow:

A. Experiment to learn your own best interval of time (out of the given sixty or ninety minutes) for a developed and coherent presentation of some ideas on a single topic. My own has turned out to be about fifteen minutes, with flexibility depending on the topic and group.

B. Give thought to what words and illustrations are pertinent to the group's work experiences.

C. Avoid technical language which has specialized meaning to an in-group in mental health.

D. Make a strong effort to involve members of the group in thinking about and reacting to the prepared material. Invite and encourage questions, discussion, and even interruptions in the initial presentation. It is important to learn skills to deal with differences of opinion and exceptions.

The purpose of the mental health educator's activity is, after all, to involve group members in thinking, reacting, and testing mental health concepts, even at the expense of omitting some material.

16. **Such thinking relates as much to private life as to work life. Should one avoid personal illustrations and references, as in consultation?**

You are correct in saying that this kind of teaching arouses re-evaluation of personal life experience. Such illustrative material encourages understanding and emotional acceptance of an idea. I think that theoretical material does need that kind of personal validation. Many points in mental health concepts have to do with attitudes. The attitudes of those studying mental health make up one of the most important areas for testing and realizing common human feelings and needs.

Mental health education is of benefit not only to caretaking groups (welfare workers, teachers, ministers, etc.), but also to lay groups such as parents in PTA groups, young people's groups, and old people's groups. You can see that in these associations personal attitudes and life experiences generally play a large part in discussion and illustration.

This leads to a definition of mental health education from a pamphlet entitled *Consultation and Education* (NIMH pamphlet 1478):

"The primary goal of mental health education is to promote positive mental health by helping people acquire knowledge, attitudes and behavior patterns that will foster and maintain their mental wellbeing . . . through a planned knowledge-building sequence of presentations and discussions."*

17. Your definition of mental health education seems rather narrow to me. The practice of community mental health is expanding in many ways, and the field includes many more kinds of activities in mental health education. NIMH's latest definition includes "training in specific job or task-related skills."** I think I prefer the broader definition.

Many practitioners in community mental health operate in this more inclusive way, making no distinction between education as a teaching-learning intellectual enterprise, and training as a teaching activity-behavioral enterprise, focusing on activity in a task. You may prefer the broader definition that includes *training* and *intellectual grasp* in the term "education."

Other kinds of activities often grouped with mental health education are:

A. Training volunteers to answer the "hot line" of a suicide prevention service.

B. Training nonpsychiatric staff to interview patients in a venereal disease clinic in order to gain fuller reports of "contacts."

C. Training nonpsychiatric admissions clerks in preliminary intake procedures for a psychiatric hospital or clinic.

D. Training personnel who hire employees for support services in a mental hospital (cooks, gardeners, etc.).

If you have taught people to grasp and think about a new idea (an intellectual enterprise) or helped people to act differently in their work because of the incorporation of some new idea (a training and consultative enterprise), it is worthwhile activity for a

*Public Health Service Publication No. 1478 (Washington, D.C.: U.S. Government Printing Office, 1966), p. 4.

**NIMH pamphlet No. 2169, 1971, "The Scope of Community Mental Health Consultation and Education," p. 21.

mental health professional. The value of a definition lies in whether it helps *the doer, the mental health professional,* to be more clear about what he is doing, and thus he may be more effective in the skills he draws into play to meet different needs and different purposes.

---

exercises for chapter 9

The size of group needed for these practice sessions varies with the specific exercise.

1. You are a staff member of a community mental health center. A call comes to you from a social worker who identifies herself as having been a member of a mental health education project you led last year under the sponsorship of the local YWCA. Three months ago she changed her job from a private family service agency to a small institution for dependent children. She says: "That place is back in the Dark Ages! You just can't imagine the way they talk to the children! They certainly need those mental health ideas from top to bottom. I'm the only one who leaves the place at five o'clock. All the rest live on the grounds. Could you give us those mental health lectures?"
   A. Begin the dialogue there.
   B. Plan your next steps.

2. You are a staff member of a mental health center whose director developed a contract with the principal of the nearby elementary school for a series of eight sessions with his twenty-eight teachers on the topic, "Child Development."
   With high commendation, the principal introduces you at the first meeting and leaves. Lightly you attempt to brush off the high praise. After a few moments of awkward silence, one teacher leans forward in her chair and says: "Tell us, doctor, what is *your* theory of child development?"
   A. Take the situation from there, with the rest of the group as the teachers.

B. The principal makes the same introduction, but sits down on an end chair, partly facing the group and partly facing you. Take the situation from there.

3. The director of your community mental health center made clear arrangements with the principal of a nearby elementary school for you to conduct eight sessions with his faculty of twenty-seven teachers on the topic, "Child Development." On the appointed day you go over a half hour early to introduce yourself to the principal and to get some idea of how he has presented the project to his teachers. The principal, however, has been busy with a delegation of parents and disengages himself only in time to take you to the room and introduce you as "a prominent psychologist whom we are fortunate to have with us to give these lectures on 'Mental Health in the Schools.'" Moving toward the door, he says, "I leave you in good hands."
   A. Begin there, with the rest of the group taking the parts of the teachers.
   B. Plan your next steps with the principal.

4. Same situation as in exercise 3. By dint of hard work in meeting initial skepticism and resistance, you have managed to evoke a fair sense of trust from most of the teachers. This is the beginning of the fourth session, and the topic for today is "The Slow Learner." After a few remarks which reflect your sympathy with the child and his frustration in coping with his world, and sympathy with his family and teachers, who need to help the child to find some ways of coping with these troubles, you comment that some parents and teachers find it difficult to accept the child's pace of learning. One teacher starts to cry softly and says: "None of you know what that means, but I do."
   What would you do? How would you carry on as the leader of the group?

5. There are in the school system special schools for children with emotional and adjustment problems called "opportunity schools." They are small in size, with ten to twelve teachers and fewer than one hundred children. Generally, the children are at least ten or eleven years old, as it is unusual to refer a child who had not shown serious problems over several years.

You have received the above information from the principal of such a school, who telephoned your community mental health center, asking your director to send someone over to give him "some mental health aid." After he has talked at some length about the school, the good quality of his teachers, and little special problems with the youngsters, you ask him how he has thought to use "some mental health aid." Hesitantly, he says: "There's one teacher here who is a troublemaker. I can't have one faculty meeting without his creating a disturbance. I can't get rid of him, and I want you to get him out of my hair!"

Continue the dialogue with the principal.

6. As a staff member of a community mental health center, you are conducting a mental health education project with the twelve teachers of grades five and six in a nearby elementary school. The topic is "Problems in Adjustment of Pre-teenagers." This is the third educational project your center has conducted with this school, and a good working relationship has developed between the school and the center. This is your seventh session of twelve meetings, planned to take place in the fall semester up to the Christmas holidays.

In this session you suddenly get a clear sense from the discussion, which has been more free and spontaneous than heretofore, that the group of twelve divides into seven older teachers, with a "status quo" stance toward schools and education, and five younger teachers, with an intense interest in change in educational methods and content.

    A. Talk for a few minutes about the implications of this split for your mental health education project.

    B. With twelve of the group acting as the teachers, conduct the rest of the session, with the purpose of making constructive use of your realization of the division in the group.

7. The director of your community mental health center has effected a good contract with the principal of the senior high school for a series of eight sessions on "Use and Abuse of Drugs," a subject of great concern to the principal and teachers. The principal has said he feels helpless and hopeless about the whole thing. He has planned to attend the meetings, and you have had

five sessions. The principal generally starts with the group but leaves or is called out within twenty minutes and sometimes returns just before closing time. You feel that this kind of attendance is a distraction in the group, and that it does not offer the principal a fair opportunity to change his attitude.

    A. Plan your next steps with the principal.

    B. How would you deal in the group with the fact of the principal's sporadic attendance? The group will take the part of the teachers. Begin the meeting.

I would try to discuss it with the group of teachers because any in-and-out attendance in a group affects the group process, and this person's in-and-out attendance is especially important because he is the principal of the school, and he feels "helpless and hopeless" about the problem. Any shift in attitude and action of the teachers might well be stymied by the principal and *they*, the teachers, would know that.

"Dealing with it in the group" does not mean organizing to act against the principal but to elicit the emotional reactions to the situation, sharing your understanding of its implications and trying to assess with the group the possible influences on this educational project.

8. As a staff member of a community mental health center, you have been conducting a mental health education project of ten sessions with a group of probation officers. The group is made up of men and women with from one to fifteen years of experience. You think the group has made a good start, and that you have done pretty well with them. At the fourth session you have an uncomfortable sense that a middle-aged woman who has had long experience in probation work is taking over the leadership of the group. You can remember feeling appreciative, even grateful, for her active contributions, which did indeed help the group to become involved in response and discussion.

    A. Try to deal with this in the group.

    B. Try to deal with the talkative woman who seems to be usurping the role of leader.

9. As a staff member of a community mental health center, you have been conducting a mental health education project in one district office of the Department of Public Social Services. There has been

a long and constructive collaboration between the two agencies for the past four or five years. You have been meeting with a group of twelve people for a planned series of ten sessions on the topic, "Dependency and Authority in a Social Context." The group is made up of two supervisors and their ten staff social workers (a pattern which has been very effective in this agency). At this fifth session, however, you realize that there are four staff workers who have made no verbal contribution from the start of this project.

Try to deal with this in the group, with twelve trainees making up the Department of Public Social Services group. Continue the session, making use of your new awareness.

10. As a staff member of a community mental health center, you have been conducting a mental health education project in an elementary school, with its twenty-five teachers, on the topic of "Factors in Non-Learning." A series of eight sessions in the fall semester had been planned with the principal and with the teachers.

By the fourth session it is evident that the teachers' discussion of concepts and ideas is definitely related to their experience with individual children in their care. Much as they are interested in the general mental health content, they say freely that their biggest concern is for help in what to do — specific ideas about how they can help the children more effectively.

Try to clarify this shift from an educational focus on general learning about "Factors in Non-Learning" to a consultative focus on "how to help specific children to make better use of the learning opportunities." This entails different responsibilities and the willingness of each teacher to present, in a more detailed way, a particular child with whom she would like some help.

/pecial Features of Mental Health Consultation with Groups

1. Although we have talked about the consultation process as occurring both with individuals and with groups of consultees, I feel as if I need to know more about some of the special features of working as a consultant with groups. Can you tell me some more about that?

Most mental health consultation today is done in groups, primarily in an effort to reach more people. In my view, a mental health consultant should be able to work with either individuals or groups, as circumstances require. Surprisingly, some professionals with years of consultation experience have worked *only* with groups.

For the mental health professional there is a special seductive quality about the process of starting a group. It is a way of establishing a place for himself in a consultee agency. However, he must still carefully plan and develop the administrative linkages necessary to effective system consultation. Moreover, the consultant should be willing to assess with the agency whether its consultation needs can best be met by meeting with individuals or groups.

129

2. **When is group consultation appropriate?**

It is appropriate when a group of consultees share a common task or closely related tasks, and when the agency prefers that consultation be in groups. Undoubtedly group consultation means a saving in time. However, we must keep in mind that reaching more people in consultation is not a substitute for working with the individual most in need.

3. **How is group consultation different from sensitivity training? Don't many consultants use sensitivity training methods in consultation?**

There is an increasing amount of confusion about this. Sensitivity training developed from working with groups of strangers: people who came from different locations and different agencies. Many sensitivity trainers refuse to accept people if they have relationships outside the group. Sensitivity training is usually oriented toward personal growth or designed to increase the participants' awareness of group behavior. It is not designed to accomplish a particular organizational task. The fact that they are strangers frees the participants to explore their feelings.

In group mental health consultation the individuals do work and live together within an already established set of rules and regulations: they are a "work family." Consultation should be done within the organizational context and should be supportive of the organizational goals and methods. The consultation experience is a part of the ongoing flow of tasks within the organization and cannot be isolated from them. Mental health consultation is meant to facilitate the tasks of the people in the organization through discussion.

4. **But aren't there people who do sensitivity training within organizational structures and with employees who are working together toward a common task?**

Some of the same group methods *are* used in organizational development consultation, which has some of the characteristics of both mental health consultation and sensitivity training. The goal is to bring about organizational change consistent with specific human and technical needs. These methods have been used more in private industry than in human service agencies, where the focus is on working with clients. The mental health consultant should be cautious about changing the balance in this way, for there is a danger of diminishing the capacity of the worker to do his job. The sensitivity approach opens questions about every aspect of the work and may reduce the concern of the individual worker for his immediate task.

Moreover, in public agencies, much of the activity is prescribed by law and regulated by code, allowing relatively small latitude for intraorganizational maneuverability. Whatever methods are used, the consultant should remember the importance of maintaining the linkages and communications with the various components of the system.

Also, organizational consultants often work within a different time framework from the mental health consultants. They conduct intensive full-time sessions for limited periods of from half a day to several days. Such intensive group meetings for a short period of time open up issues of importance. The organization then has an extended period to translate what has been revealed into its operation.

By contrast, mental health consultation is an ongoing process which is only one aspect of a total community program. The usual consultee agency's concern is with the immediate services offered to needy human beings. Such agencies have an ongoing need for consultation with a representative of the mental health program in order to serve clients more effectively.

5. **On the whole, how much of a mental health consultant's group effort are process-oriented and how much task-oriented?**

That is a crucial decision for the consultant: when to focus on the intragroup issues and when to focus on the specific tasks of the consultees. Our view is that the consultant should maintain primary focus on the tasks. How much process discussion he admits and encourages in the consultation is an individual matter, for different emphases are certainly possible within our models. The principal concern, I believe, is that the consultant should remain cognizant of the fact that his purpose is to facilitate the task effectiveness of the workers.

This means that the consultant should be ready to intervene where the process does not seem to be supporting the task. The consultant, of course, hopes to leave the consultees better able to do their jobs than before the session.

If the consultant begins to sense that something is happening in the group to undermine the sense of confidence or competence of a member or members, he will probably wish to redirect the focus in such a way that the group will once again work toward its common goal.

For example, sometimes a group will begin to use consultation as a session for complaint against the organization. A consultant may feel, rightly, that a certain amount of such candor is useful. However, such a complaint session may become self-perpetuating. Implicit in the consultees' complaints is the expectation something will be done about them. The consultant, however, usually has neither a contract nor the power to do much in this area. Thus, the group members may leave more dissatisfied than they were before the consultation, feeling that they cannot do their jobs because of administrative and organization obstructions.

The consultant will wish to refocus the discussion onto their tasks. Of course he should acknowledge the importance of their comments and the problems discussed, but he should then try to restate the consultation goal and to examine how, within the constraints, the given job can be done best.

If the organizational and administrative issues are important, the consultant cannot ignore them. He should keep this knowledge for a time when he can use it constructively. With the group's permission, he may later review what he has learned about the administrative problems with the administrative officer who authorized his contract. If their relationship has matured and trust has developed, this can be done without disruption.

The administration may then use the consultant to seek ways of dealing with these problems. For example, the contract may be renegotiated to include some means for working on them. Until this is done the consultant must be careful not to step beyond what he has agreed to do.

In another example of changing focus, one of the consultees may begin to see himself as the problem in a given case. He may see himself as being so neurotically impaired that he is unable to do his job. While in psychotherapy this might be constructive, in the consultation situation it probably will limit his work ability even further.

6. **If that does occur, how should the consultant handle it?**

    First, the consultant must acknowledge that the focus has shifted in this situation from a work problem to a personality problem. He should reassure the consultee and the group of consultees that it is all right to have such feelings. Then he can focus on what positive use may be made of them; for example, he may say that experiencing such feelings may allow the consultee to understand more about the problems experienced by his client. The consultant should then try to return to the client focus and see what can be done.

    In yet another example, the group may become increasingly critical of the work of one of its members. Again, the consultant should acknowledge the positive elements of this criticism: the desire for improvement within the group. However, the consultant should then in some way try to restore the group's sense of purpose in working toward a common goal. He may do this by a process observation such as, "What in this case causes our group to become so self-critical?"

7. **You seem overly protective of the consultee. It is as though you don't think he can handle a frank discussion of feelings. I have more confidence in a person's capacity to deal openly with feelings. I don't think it is necessary to be so cautious.**

    There are legitimate differences in points of view about this. What is important here is to recognize the task-oriented quality of consultation and the limited nature of the consultant's contract. Certainly the consultant must not be afraid of the consultee's feelings and he must be open to deal with whatever the consultee brings up, but he must also keep a perspective consistent with his task. In the human services field the element of personal feeling occupies such an important place that the boundary between a consultee's professional needs and his personal needs becomes vague. In our model the aim is to increase the consultee's ability to do his job. The consultant's role is a temporary one, and thereby different from that of the psychotherapist, who may take the position that the patient will have to get worse before he can get better. The consultee, however, is working "on the firing line" with people in need. It is our goal that he be able to help them effectively without declaring a moratorium until he "gets better."

8. **In my work with people as a clinician, I have learned to be an expressive and open person about my feelings, and that is what I want of those with whom I work. I am concerned that the model you present is too constricting.**

   How much of personal feelings and motivations becomes a part of the consultation process is an individual matter for the consultant and the consultees. I would emphasize the importance of keeping focused on the task, keeping the organizational perspectives, and implying no more than one can actually do as a consultant. As long as feelings and motivations are kept constructively within this framework, the consultant is doing his job.

9. **I think I can see that. I accept the concept you have expressed of treating the consultee as a competent equal, and I understand the importance of not leaving him less able to do his job than before the consultation. It seems to me, however, that the consultee needs to use *all* of himself, including his feelings, in order to do his job.**

   I agree entirely. The attitudinal blocks, theme interferences, and stereotyping of the consultee are the result of his inability to perform as a whole human being utilizing all of his resources. His feelings have gotten out of hand in some way so that he can neither see the client as he is nor hear him accurately. His vision and hearing are clouded by an emotionally charged idea. Our goal is to restore his wholeness so that he can perform his job with his full effectiveness. What our model provides is a way of doing this while still maintaining the focus on his job and treating the consultee as someone competent to do the job. Certainly feelings are admitted and encouraged, but they must be seen in the context of the model we have discussed.

   Often the observations that the consultant makes are, in a sense, giving the consultee or the consultees permission to have feelings within the job context. That is, the consultee is told that it is understandable that the unwilling client should provoke his frustration or his anger since he, as a professional who has a job to do, is conscientious in wanting to fulfill that job.

10. **Can you discuss other ways of keeping the focus in a group when it seems to be concentrating on the criticism of one consultee or an exposure of psychopathology?**

One way is to give a short discussion of the principles involved in the case under discussion. A short discourse on crisis intervention, personality development, or community resources will help to return the group to its focus and at the same time remove an element that might prove to be destructive.

Another way is to relate a personal experience involving similar clients. This is like the parable method described earlier; it allows the consultant to convey a message that it is acceptable to have negative feelings, that one does not need to know instantly what to do, or that there is more to be seen in the case.

11. **Can you mention some ways in which a *group* of consultees rather than an individual can be used with special advantage in dealing with a consultation problem?**

We have talked previously about the importance of confirming the group's feelings about a common task. With a group, additional competence can also be brought to bear in solving a particular problem.

In group theme interferences, there is sometimes a particular stereotype shared by most of the people who work in an agency. This problem can best be dealt with in a group, which together can examine what might be done in a case which might otherwise seem hopeless.

Where there is an individual theme interference, other members of the group may bring their own perceptions to bear on widening the individual's understanding of the case. They can serve then as allies to the consultant in examining the case material and in providing information which will tend to broaden the picture so that the bad outcome is not seen as inevitable.

12. **If an individual consultee is presenting within a group, does the consultant then try to get the other group members to participate in the discussion?**

Yes. He would wish to invite them, both to learn what they know about the case and to determine if they have had similar problems. He will get a sense of the group issues as they relate to the individual consultee. Sometimes there will be members of the "work family" who share responsibility for working with a client. In such a situation the common problem or the interlinking problem can be explored.

13. **I can see that in a "work family" there might be some very strong intragroup tensions. How can one deal with those?**

Again the consultant must decide how much to stay with the task and how much to explore the process. My own inclination is to keep the focus on the task so as to avoid the expression of group tensions which cannot be resolved within the group. Focus on the task gives the group a sense of unity. The consultant, of course, may perceive certain causes of group tension and may seek to alter these as we discussed earlier when talking about the parallel process. Even so, much can be accomplished simply by staying with the common task.

14. **From what you have said, I gather that you favor having supervisors and workers in the same group, and perhaps even administrators.**

This is one of the options open to the consultant. In large part, the decision may depend upon the structure of the organization and what its members want. If there are administrators, supervisors, and workers in the same group, the workers may have serious problems in expressing their feelings about the case situation. The group may become stratified in the same way that the organization is stratified. One of the advantages of consultation is that the consultant is not responsible to administration in the way that the supervisor is, so that his consultees can discuss material that might be precluded elsewhere.

On the positive side, if all levels of the organization are represented in the consultee group, meaningful organizational change in meeting a client's needs or doing a task may be facilitated. The decision-making forces are available if needed. So there are advantages in either arrangement, depending on the circumstances.

15. **If a group is very slow to start in discussing problems, what techniques can a consultant use?**

Sometimes a consultant will meet a group that is very reserved and cautious about saying anything. Of course, he should immediately be alert to what this tells him about the organization. The usual means for starting a discussion is to inquire about what kinds of cases or problems the workers face. This may produce little response since it is asking the workers, in effect, to show their weaknesses. Particularly among human service workers, there is a much greater desire to be helpful than to be helped.

A consultant may use this desire positively, however, in getting consultation started. He can, for example, ask the group to describe one of their successes in improving a client's mental health. This may prove a more egosyntonic task to those who see themselves as helpers. This is also in keeping with our model of respecting the consultee as competent. Soon, the consultees will begin to feel comfortable in sharing some of the cases that are not going so well — but only after they have established themselves as competent.

16. **How is it decided who will be the presenting consultee in a particular session?**

This is done in various ways. One means is to assign people in rotation and ask them to present protocols in writing in advance of the discussion. My own preference, however, is to try to develop a climate of spontaneity and trust, so that whoever has something pressing can bring it up.

The highly organized assignment, with protocol plan, is almost the opposite of what we discussed in the above question where no one has anything to say. These represent problems of the beginning phase and are part of the consultee's efforts to find out what is safe and how far he can trust the consultant.

---

exercises for chapter 10

1. The consultant has begun to meet with a group of eight elementary schoolteachers. At first he observed the group to be very reticent, and when no one volunteered to present a case he elected to do some mental health education. He spent the first three sessions talking about community resources for referral and developmental crises in elementary school youngsters. He hoped that this might serve as an "ice-breaker," but now in the fourth session he asks again if anyone has work problems to discuss and

there is no response. Reenact the scene to this point and then continue the consultation session.

2. A consultant has been meeting with a group of twelve ministers at their request. They are extremely enthusiastic about the consultation and come each week filled with issues and problems for discussion. As soon as one of the consultees begins to discuss a case, another is reminded of one of his cases. A third interrupts to bring up an administrative issue, which reminds a fourth of a personal experience, and so on. The consultant has to fight to get a word in. His concern is that while there is a lot of discussion, it is largely "free association," so that by the end of the session there has been no focus. At the end of the third session a couple of side comments suggest to him that some group members are beginning to feel that the sessions are more fun than useful. He decides that he should probably take some action in the next session. At the beginning of the next session, the fourth, the group begins as before, very chatty and talkative but unfocused. A case that is brought up is immediately diverted by another comment. Reenact this scene and then continue the dialogue as the consultant attempts to focus the consultation.

3. A group of eight probation officers have been meeting with a consultant for four sessions. They have been very expressive and the consultant has had the impression that the consultation has been going well. He feels that they have focused on some important cases and he has seen some progress in both individual members and the group. In the fourth session one of the members says, "After the last session I was talking to Charlie and we thought that what the group really ought to be doing is having sensitivity training. If we can understand ourselves better and deal with some of our problems we could help people we work with more, don't you think?" As he says this he looks around the room and two or three of the others nod agreement. Reenact the scene to this point and then continue the dialogue with the consultant.

4. The consultant has been meeting with school nurses from a variety of elementary schools. The group varies in size from seven to ten. They have met for one school term and are beginning the second. The consultant has had positive feelings about the sessions

and the comments from the consultees suggest that they agree. Until recently, the discussions have been case-centered. From time to time, administrative problems beyond the control of the nurses have been brought up, but after some discussion the group has gone on to case-centered discussions. In the last two sessions there has been a change. The group has begun to complain about some recent administrative fiats having to do with working hours, sabbaticals, leaves, and assignments to schools. The consultant hoped that this would diminish and they would be able to get back to the case consultation, but this has not been the case. Instead, dissatisfaction has steadily increased as the group complains impotently about what is being done to them. This session begins the same way. The consultant feels he must try to make the consultation experience a constructive one. Reenact this scene and then continue the session.

5. The same group as above begins the session by saying, "We've talked about these administrative problems that are really interfering with our work. Several of us talked between sessions and we have a request of you. We would like you to see if you can't get some of these things straightened out: particularly the issue about our being transferred from school to school each term. It never allows us to get acquainted with the children adequately. Will you take this up with the school superintendent and tell him how important it is?" Reenact this scene and then continue the dialogue with the consultant.

6. A group of school nurses working in elementary schools have been meeting with a consultant for one term and are about halfway through the second term. There are seven to ten members in each session. The consultant has been impressed with their interest, competence, and use of the consultation sessions. He has also observed that there appear to be two factions in the group. Half the group consists of nurses who have been with the school system an average of twenty years. The other half is made up of young nurses who have been with the school only a couple of years. They sit on opposite sides of the table and tend to disagree when issues come up. So far, however, this has not presented a special problem to the consultation.

   One of the young nurses begins the session by talking about a young fifth grade boy who is absent a great deal and who, when present, falls asleep in class. His teacher usually then sends him to the school nurse. She has tried to talk with him to find out what the problem is. She has wondered if there is anything in the home that makes it difficult for him to sleep there and she has also wondered if drugs might be a problem, as they are with some of the other boys in his class. Immediately after school, a few days ago, she decided that she would walk home with the boy and find out first-hand what was going on, if she could. When she arrived with the student at his apartment in a dilapidated housing tract, the boy went around back and she knocked on the front door. The boy's mother would talk to the nurse only through a crack. She was very hostile, would give her no information, would not let her in the house and told her to "mind your own business." The nurse was very upset about this and sees this boy as being in serious trouble. She raised the question of what she might do. Immediately, one of the older nurses says, "In the first place, you should not have made that home visit. This should have been referred to the welfare and attendance officer or to the vice principal. You are stepping out of line." One of the young nurses immediately responded, "That's the biggest trouble with our schools and our nursing program. You old fuddy-duddies are so preoccupied with following the rules that you never help anybody." Members immediately leap to the defense of their respective sides, all talking at once and very angry. Reenact this scene and then pick up the discussion at this point with the consultant.

7. A consultant has been working with the Department of Public Social Services for over a year. He meets with Protective Services workers in a group that varies in size from ten to fifteen. As the group has matured and become more expressive, he has found himself dealing more and more with theme interference issues.

   On this occasion a young worker, who has been a member of the group for some time and whom the consultant has observed to be sensitive, thoughtful, and an effective worker, presents the case of a mother of three illegitimate children. The problem she presents is that the mother has spoken of wanting to get rid of the children. She says that she cannot stand to have them around and that they interfere with her life, making it impossible to get a job or to meet people. Recently, she has been very depressed and has expressed both suicidal and homicidal wishes.*

The worker is very distressed about this and appears herself to be somewhat depressed. She says, "Any mother is better than a substitute mother, no matter how bad she is." She goes on to say that she has had a very good working relationship with this client and she hates to see her "ruin her life" and that of the children at this time.

The consultee is very free and open in her discussion of the problem and the consultant begins to detect a theme interference having to do with the feeling that her own relationship with the client is threatened. The consultant hypothesizes that the worker's panic and depression may be over the fact that should the children be given up she would no longer have occasion to meet with the client, who has become important to her. He further begins to note that the data from the case suggest that, indeed, both the children and the mother might be better off should they be given up for adoption as the mother wishes.

Recognizing the worker's feelings in this matter, the consultant begins to work carefully, examining the data of the case, attempting to deal with the theme. Abruptly, one of the other workers breaks in and says, "The problem in this case is not the client but you (the worker); you don't want to let her go. The mother is quite willing to give up those children but you're afraid that you won't be able to work with the mother again."

The worker appears demolished and stunned. She starts to speak a couple of times but then just shakes her head, seemingly in agreement with the statement. The rest of the group is momentarily silent. Reenact this scene and then continue the dialogue. The consultant's task is to figure out what to do at this point.

8. A consultant has been meeting on a weekly basis with a group of junior high schoolteachers. This is the eighth session with a group of seven teachers. The group has been lively and the consultant has felt that the case-centered discussion has gone well. He has been aware of some theme interference in some members, which, however, he believes to be lessening with successive cases.

*Case adapted from presentation by Alexander S. Rogawski, M.D. at Center for Training in Community Psychiatry, Los Angeles, 1970.

All of the members of the group have presented cases except one. She appears to be little older than the students she is teaching, and is in fact much younger than the other members of the consultee group. She has been the subject of much "kidding." The references are always to her youth and immaturity. Although the consultant has thought, on occasion, that the barbs were a little sharp, this teacher seemed almost pleased with the joking. The consultant has hypothesized that she is the group's scapegoat.

In this session she begins to speak for the first time. She says, "I just don't know what to do. I'm afraid it's more than I can handle." She goes on to say that there are a couple of boys in her class who refuse to follow her instructions. They make light of them and show her no respect. Recently, she had started discussion of a class project and one of the boys got up and said that he didn't feel like doing that project, and that he had other things to do that were more interesting to him. One of the other teachers in the consultee group said, "Maybe he was interested in a date with you." The others laughed loudly. The young teacher smiled, but this time without mirth. Reenact this scene and then continue the dialogue as the consultant attempts to deal with this issue.

9. A consultant has been meeting with a group of ministers of various Protestant denominations. The group started with about fifteen members and has gradually consolidated to eight regulars. They are now in their twelfth session. The consultant has enjoyed the experience and has felt that the group was very responsive to his efforts. The discussions have been case-centered, with all of the members quite active. On this occasion one of the younger ministers says that he would like to talk about something that has been bothering him for some time. He says that he has found that in his pastoral counseling, a number of homosexuals have started coming to him. He wonders if he has done something that has caused them to seek him out. In addition, he finds himself attracted to some of the men and has been wondering if he is suited for the ministry. He feels he cannot objectively talk with men who have homosexual problems. The whole thing was precipitated when a young man whom he had seen once came back and asked the minister if he would be willing to see him on a regular basis to counsel with him about his homosexual problem.

One of the older members of the group says that it does

appear that his emotional problems may be too great a burden in his ministry and that he should perhaps think of leaving. Two of the other members immediately respond that it seems like a perfectly human response and that he should not think of leaving the ministry. Reenact this scene and then continue the dialogue with the consultant at this point.

10. A consultant has been meeting with a group of public health nurses. This is the sixth session. The group has been very orderly. When one person is presenting the others are silent and the discussion is only between the consultee and the consultant. The consultant feels that he would like to have more group participation.

In this session one of the nurses from the Well Baby Clinic says that she would like to discuss the problem of a young mother who is only sixteen years old. She seems quite helpless, attends the clinic faithfully, asks many questions and often tries to stay longer in order to talk to the nurse. The nurse says that she thinks this client may be looking at her as a mother figure. She doesn't know what to do about it or how to go about understanding it further. Reenact this scene and then continue the dialogue as the consultant tries to involve the group in the discussion of this case.

11. A consultant has met with a group of probation officers for four sessions. The group is made up of six deputy probation officers and two supervisors. The consultant has noted that the supervisors stringently control the meetings so that when a worker presents a case, one of the supervisors often will give what sounds like a "prescription" for what should be done. Then he will turn to the consultant and say, "Isn't that right, doctor?"

In this, the fifth session, the consultant is determined to try to involve the group more openly in discussion. One of the officers begins to present the case of a sixteen-year-old juvenile who has been arrested twice for "joy riding." The interesting thing about it is that the boy's father is the owner of a used car lot. The officer says he feels that the consultant might be able to help him understand what's going on and to help the boy. Reenact this scene and then continue the dialogue with the probation officer presenting. The consultant sees this as a good opportunity to involve the whole group in a freer discussion.

Postscript

This primer and study guide has been organized so that an individual or a group may use it for educational purposes to develop or increase skills in mental health consultation. It can be used as a textbook and as the basis for a weekly study group. In the latter case, one chapter a week can serve as the text for discussion; following that, exercises and simulations can be used to illustrate the text and deepen the cognitive understanding of it.

Within this agenda there are a number of variations possible. One of the most useful is to include actual consultation experiences of the members of the study group. Presumably, some or all of the members of a study group have been engaged in some phase of mental health consultation. To select some nodal issues or problems as the focus of a study group will serve as an important method of teaching.

These live experiences, presented by members of the study group, can be handled in a number of ways. However, our experience is that certain guidelines help to keep the study group from deteriorating into a nonproductive speculative case conference which avoids practical issues. Another problem may develop if the experiences described are subjected to an unstructured discussion: a sharply critical stance may be taken by the members of the group not presenting. It becomes a "sniping" session in which each member attempts to outdo the others in making the most acidulous observation. Soon, understandably, there is a diminished enthusiasm for presenting a case.

One useful method we have found is to structure the presentation of the experience as an analogue to the mental health consultation process. That is, the group members function as consultants to the consultant describing his experience with one or more consultees. The consultant who presents, thus, has the experience of being a consultee while describing his own experience as a consultant.

Under these conditions members of the group attempt to be constructive and useful to the presenter. They should employ all of the principles described in the preceding text: they will wish to strengthen the consultee's role identification, leave him with a greater sense of confidence and competence, and examine the content in the context of mental health issues rather than judgmentally.

Following this presentation of a consultation experience, the group can evaluate whether the comments made to the presenter were constructive or not. Thus, there is a simultaneous double level consideration of the consultation process which tends to emphasize the ways in which basic human experience transcends the limits of the roles of consultant and consultee.

Another useful method for structuring discussion in the study group is to reenact the experience described with members of the group in the various roles described. This allows the participants to have not only a cognitive but an emotional sense of the experience. Following this, discussion can be based on the data of actual experience.

The text and exercises can be covered in a period of ten to twelve weeks in a study group. In learning a complicated new skill like mental health consultation, members may often wish to continue to study. Thus it may be profitable to extend a study group beyond this initial period by continuing to draw upon the participants' live consultation experiences in the way described above. If there are not enough live experiences for study, the exercises described in the body of the primer can be utilized over and over again to provide live data. One can learn an almost endless amount from serial simulations of a consultation experience.

Experience at the Center for Training in Community Psychiatry in Los Angeles and other centers offering courses in mental health consultation suggests that a period of nine months to a year in weekly study is adequate to learning the basic skills of mental health consultation. The first ten to twelve weeks should be devoted to the utilization of the primer and the exercises. As previously suggested, focus can continue with live experiences or further simulations of the exercises.

Social change continues at an ever-increasing rate. The organizations to which consultants offer services are caught in this change, thereby requiring that a consultant be ever alert to new demands upon him. Changes in specialized programs for the provision of services also make necessary from time to time a restructuring of the immediate goals and purposes of consultation. It is, therefore, advantageous even beyond the initial period of study of mental health consultation to meet periodically with a group of peers and a teacher, if possible, to review the changes which have occurred in experiences. This will allow for a retailoring of what the consultant has learned to meet new situations in his role as a consultant and the new needs of consultee organizations.

At this Center we have found such continuing study groups or periodic reorientation groups to be extremely valuable. As mental health professionals we can hardly be expected to provide meaningful and responsive services to people who are the victims of the ambiguities produced by change, if we ourselves do not have a forum in which we can deal with the ambiguities faced by us in our helping roles.

Bibliography

introduction

Bellak, L. (ed.) *Handbook of Community Psychiatry and Community Mental Health*. New York: Grune and Stratton, 1963.

Berlin, I. N. *Learning Mental Health Consultation: History and Problems, Mental Hygiene*, 48, 2 (April 1964), 257-66.

Caplan, G. *Concepts of Mental Health and Consultation: Their Application in Public Health Social Work*. Washington, D.C.: U.S. Department of Health, Education, and Welfare, 1959.

Caplan, G. *Principles of Preventative Psychiatry*. New York: Basic Books, 1964.

Caplan, G. *The Theory and Practice of Mental Health Consultation*. New York: Basic Books, 1970.

Coleman, J. V. "Psychiatric Consultation in Casework Agencies," *American Journal of Orthopsychiatry*, 17, 3 (July 1947), 533-39.

Leighton, D. C., et al. *The Character of Danger*. New York: Basic Books, 1963.

Lewin, K. "Group Decision and Social Change," *Readings in Social Psychology*, G. E. Swanson, T. M. Newcomb, E. L. Hartley (eds.). New York: Holt, Rinehart and Winston, Inc., 1958.

147

Maddux, J. F. "Psychiatric Consultation in a Public Welfare Agency," *American Journal of Orthopsychiatry*, 20, 4 (October 1950), 754-64.

Mayo, E. *Human Problems of an Industrial Civilization*. New York: Viking Press, 1960.

Mendel, W. M. and Solomon, P. *The Psychiatric Consultation*. New York: Grune and Stratton, 1968.

Rapoport, L. "The Theory and Practice of Mental Health Consultation by Gerald Caplan." Book Review, *Social Service Review*, June 1971, 223-24.

Roethlisberger, F. and Dickson, W. *Management and The Worker*. Cambridge, Mass.: Harvard University Press, 1939.

Rogers, C. *Counseling and Psychotherapy*. Boston: Houghton Mifflin, 1942.

Rogers, C. and Roethlisberger, F. "Barriers and Gateways to Communication," *Harvard Bus. Rev.*, 30 (1952), 28-34.

Schwartz, D. A. and Doran, S. M. "The No-Patient Hour," *International Psychiatry Clinics*, 3, 4 (Winter 1967), 119-37.

Srole, L., et al. *Mental Health in the Metropolis: The Midtown Manhattan Study*. New York: McGraw-Hill, 1962.

Susselman, Sam "The Role of the Psychiatrist in a Probation Agency," *Focus*, 29 (March 1950), 33.

Taylor, F. *Scientific Management*. New York: Harper and Row, 1911.

Weber, M. *The Theory of Social and Economic Organization*. Talcott Parsons (ed.), A. M. Henderson and T. Parsons (trans.). New York: Oxford University Press, 1947.

Zilboorg, G. *History of Medical Psychology*. New York: W. W. Norton Press, 1967.

chapter 2

Berlin, I. N. "Learning Mental Health Consultation History and Problems," *Mental Hygiene*, 48, 2 (April 1964), 257-66.

Bindman, A. J. "Mental Health Consultation: Theory and Practice," *Journal of Consulting Psychology*, 23, 6 (1959), 473-82.

Caplan, G. "Definition of Mental Health Consultation," Chapter 2, *The Theory and Practice of Mental Health Consultation*. New York: Basic Books, 1970.

Caplan, G. "Types of Mental Health Consultation," *American Journal of Orthopsychiatry*, 33, 3 (1963), 470-81.

Haylett, C. H. and Rapoport, L. "Mental Health Consultation." In L. Bellak (ed.) *Handbook of Community Psychiatry and Community Mental Health*. New York: Grune and Stratton, 1964, pp. 319-39.

Kazanjian, V., Stein, S., Weinberg, W. L. *An Introduction to Mental Health Consultation*. U. S. Public Health Service Publication No. 922, Public Health Monograph No. 69. Washington, D.C.: U.S. Government Printing Office, 1962.

Lippitt, R. "Dimensions of the Consultant's Job," *Journal of Social Issues,* 15, 2 (1959), 5-12.

Loeb, M. B. "Concerns and Methods of Mental Health Consultation," *Hospital and Community Psychiatry,* (April 1968), 111-13.

U. S. Dept. HEW. *The Comprehensive Community Mental Health Centers Program Grants for Construction and Staffing.* Washington, D.C.: U.S. Government Printing Office, 1969.

chapter 3

Caplan, G. "Developing a Consultation Program in a Community," Chapter 3, *The Theory and Practice of Mental Health Consultation.* New York: Basic Books, 1970.

Caplan, G. "Building Relationships with a Consultee Institution," Chapter 4, *The Theory and Practice of Mental Health Consultation.* New York: Basic Books, 1970.

Gaupp, P. G. "Authority Influence and Control in Consultation," *Community Mental Health Journal,* 2, 3 (1966), 205-10.

Haylett, C. H. "Evolution of Indirect Services." In H. R. Lamb, D. Heath, and J. J. Downing (eds.), *Handbook of Community Mental Health Practice.* San Francisco: Jossey-Bass, 1969, pp. 289-304.

Haylett, C. H. "Issues of Indirect Services." In H. Lamb, D. Heath and J. J. Downing (eds.), *Handbook of Community Mental Health Practice.* San Francisco: Jossey-Bass, 1969, pp. 305-321.

Papanek, G. O. "Dynamics of Community Consultation," *Archives of General Psychiatry.* 19 (August 1968), 189-96.

chapter 4

Argyris, C. "Explorations in Consulting-Client Relationships," *Human Organization,* 20, 3 (1961), 121-33.

Gibb, J. R. "The Role of the Consultant," *The Journal of Social Issues.* 15, 2 (1959), 1-4.

Stringer, L. A. "Consultation: Some Expectations, Principles and Skills," *Social Work,* 6, 3 (1961), 85-90.

chapter 5

Caplan, G. "Building Relationships with a Consultee Institution," Chapter 4, *The Theory and Practice of Mental Health Consultation.* New York: Basic Books, 1970.

Caplan, G. "Building the Relationship with the Consultee," Chapter 5, *The Theory and Practice of Mental Health Consultation.* New York: Basic Books, 1970.

Glidewell, J. C. "The Entry Problem in Consultation," *The Journal of Social Issues.* 15, 2 (1959), 51-59.

Mannino, F. V. "Developing Consultation Relationships with Community Agents," *Mental Hygiene.* 48 (1964), 356-62.

chapter 6

Caplan, G. "Client-Centered Case Consultation," Chapter 6, *The Theory and Practice of Mental Health Consultation.* New York: Basic Books, 1970.

Caplan, G. "Consultee-Centered Case Consultation," Chapter 7, *The Theory and Practice of Mental Health Consultation.* New York: Basic Books, 1970.

Green, R. "The Consultant and the Consultation Process," *Child Welfare Journal of the Child Welfare League of America, Inc.* 44, 8 (October 1965), 425-30.

chapter 7

Ekstein, R. and Wallerstein, R. S. "Supervisor and Student-Therapist and Patient—The Parallel Process," *The Teaching and Learning of Psychotherapy.* London: Imago, 1958, pp. 177-196.

chapter 8

Berlin, I. N. "The Theme in Mental Health Consultation Sessions," *American Journal of Orthopsychiatry.* 30, 4 (1960), 827-82.

Caplan, G. "Techniques of Theme Interference Reduction," Chapter 8, *The Theory and Practice of Mental Health Consultation.* New York: Basic Books, 1970.

Festinger, L. *Theory of Cognitive Dissonance.* Stanford University Press, 1957.

Frank, J. D. *Persuasion and Healing.* Baltimore, Md.: Johns Hopkins Press, 1961.

Rogawski, A. S. "Teaching Consultation Techniques in a Community Agency," in Mendell and Solomon (eds.), *The Psychiatric Consultation.* New York: Grune and Stratton, 1968.

Singh, R. K. J. *Community Mental Health Consultation and Crisis Intervention.* William Tarnower and Ronald Chen (eds.), Berkeley, Calif.: Book People, 1971.

chapter 9

Berlin, I. N. "Mental Health Consultation in Schools as a Means of Communicating Mental Health Principles," *Journal of the American Academy of Child Psychiatry.* 1, 4 (1962), 671-79.

Goldston, S. E. "Mental Health Education in a Community Mental Health Center," *American Journal of Public Health.* 58, 4 (1968), 693-99.

U. S. Department of Health, Education, and Welfare, Public Health Service, National Institute of Mental Health. *Consultation and Education, A Service of the Community Mental Health Center.* Washington, D.C.: Public Health Service Publication No. 1478.

U. S. Department of Health, Education, and Welfare, Public Health Service, National Institute of Mental Health. *The Scope of Community Mental Health: Consultation and Education,* prepared by Beryce W. MacLennan, et al. Washington, D.C.: Public Health Service Publication No. 2169.

chapter 10

Benne, K. D. "Some Ethical Problems in Group and Organizational Consultation," *The Journal of Social Issues,* 15, 2 (1969), 60-67.

Parker, B. *Psychiatric Consultation for Non-Psychiatric Professional Workers.* Public Health Monograph, No. 53. Washington, D.C.: U.S. Department of Health, Education, and Welfare, 1958.

Rowitch, J. "Group Consultation With School Personnel," *Hospital and Community Psychiatry,* 19, 8 (August 1968), 261-66.

Spielberger, C. and Eisdorfer, C. "Mental Health Consultation with Groups," *Community Mental Health Journal,* 1, 2 (1965), 127-34.

Subject Area:

disaster

Muhich, D. F., et al. "Professional Deployment in the Mental Health Disaster, The Range Mental Health Center," *Community Mental Health Journal.* 1, 2 (1965), 205-07.

evaluation

Behavior Science Corporation, Washington, D.C. (and Panorama City, Los Angeles). *A Study of the Theory and Practice of: Mental Health Consultation as Provided to Child Care Agencies Throughout the United States.* Washington, D.C.: National Institute of Mental Health, 1970.

MacLennan, B. W., Montgomery, S. L., and Stern, E. G. *The Analysis and Evaluation of the Consultation Component in a Community Mental Health Center.* Laboratory Paper Number 36. Adelphi, Md.: Mental Health Study Center, National Institute of Mental Health, July 1970.

Mannino, F. V., and Shore, M. F. *Consultation Research in Mental Health and Related Fields: A Critical Review of the Literature.* Public Health Monograph Number 79. Washington, D.C.: U.S. Department of Health, Education, and Welfare, Public Health Service.

Singh, R. K. J. Evaluation of a Program of Community Mental Health. Working Paper. Berkeley, 1969, 16 pages.

job corps

Caplan, G., Macht, L. B., and Wolf, A. B. *Manual for Mental Health Professionals Participating in the Job Corps Program.* Office of Economic Opportunity (JCH 330-A), May 1969. 69 pages.

Macht, L. B., et al. "Mental Health in the Job Corps: An Exploration of the Role of the Mental Health Worker in Programs of Education and Training," *Community Mental Health Journal.* 5, 5 (1969), 367-81.

law enforcement and probation

Berlin, I. N. "Mental Health Consultation with Juvenile Probation Department," *Crime and Delinquency.* January 1964, pp. 67-73.

Newman, L. E. "Consultation with Police on Human Relations Training," *American Journal of Psychiatry.* 126, 10 (April 1970), 65-73.

new organizations

Sheldon, A. "On Consulting to New, Changing, or Innovative Organizations," *Community Mental Health Journal,* 7, 1 (1971), 62-71.

public health

Maddux, J. F. "Consultation in Public Health," *American Journal of Public Health.* 45, 7 (July 1955), 1424-30.

public welfare and children

Bernard, V. W. "Psychiatric Consultation with Special Reference to Adoption Practice," *Casework Papers.* 1954.

Maddux, J. F. "Psychiatric Consultation in a Public Welfare Agency," *The American Journal of Orthopsychiatry.* 20, 4 (October 1950), 754-64.

Murphy, L. B. "The Consultant in a Day-Care Center for Deprived Children," *Children.* 15, 3 (1968), 97-102.

Nitzberg, H., and Kahn, M. W. "Consultations with Welfare Workers in a Mental Health Clinic," *Social Work.* 7, 3 (1962), 84-92.

Scheidlinger, S. and Sarcka, A. "A Mental Health Consultation: Education Program with Group Service Agencies in a Disadvantaged Community." Paper presented at the American Orthopsychiatric Association Meeting, Chicago, 1968.

U. S. Department of Health, Education, and Welfare. *Mental Health Consultation to Programs for Children: A Review of Data Collected from Selected U. S. Sites.* Public Health Service Publication No. 2066. Washington, D.C.: U. S. Government Printing Office, 1970.

Williams, M. "The Problem Profile Technique in Consultation," *Social Work.* July 1971, pp. 52-59.

rural communities

Libo, L. M. and Griffith, C. R. "Developing Mental Health Programs in Areas Lacking Professional Facilities: The Community Consultant Approach in New Mexico," *Community Mental Health Journal.* 2, 2 (1966), 163-69.

Maddux, J. F. "Psychiatric Consultation in a Rural Setting," *American Journal of Orthopsychiatry.* 23, 4 (October 1953), 775-84.

Spielberger, C. "A Mental Health Consultation Program in a Small Community with Limited Professional Mental Health Resources," in E. L. Cown, E. A. Gardner, and M. Zax (eds.), *Emergent Approaches to Mental Health Problems.* New York: Appleton-Century-Crofts, 1967, 214-38.

schools and nursery schools

Berkovitz, I. H. "Mental Health Consultation to School Personnel: Attitudes of School Administrators and Consultant Priorities," *Journal of School Health,* 40, 7 (September 1970), 348-54.

Berkovitz, I. H. "Varieties of Mental Health Consultation for School Personnel," *Journal of Secondary Education.* 45, 3 (March 1970).

Berlin, I. N. "Some Learning Experiences as Psychiatric Consultant in the Schools," *Mental Hygiene.* 40, 2 (April 1956), 215-36.

Berlin, I. N. "Consultation and Special Education," in Irving Philips (ed.), *Prevention and Treatment of Mental Retardation.* New York: Basic Books, Inc., 1966.

Berlin, I. N. "Preventive Aspects of Mental Health Consultation to Schools," *Mental Hygiene.* 51, 1 (January 1967), 34-40.

Berlin, I. N. "Mental Health Consultation for School Social Workers: A Conceptual Model," *Community Mental Health Journal.* 5, 4 (1969), 280-88.

Latimer, N., et al. *The Protection and Promotion of Mental Health in Schools.* Bethesda, Md.: U. S. Department of Health, Education, and Welfare, National Institute of Mental Health, 1964.

Newman, R. G. *Psychological Consultation in the Schools.* New York: Basic Books, 1967.

Parker, B. "Some Observations on Psychiatric Consultation with Nursery School Teachers," *Mental Hygiene.* 46, 4 (October 1962), 559-66.

Rowitch, J. "Group Consultation with School Personnel," *Hospital and Community Psychiatry.* 19, 8 (August 1968), 261-66.

others

Mannino, F. V. *Consultation in Mental Health and Related Fields: A Reference Guide.* Chevy Chase, Md.: National Institute of Mental Health, 1969.

Index